EQUINE DENTISTRY

A PRACTICAL GUIDE

EQUINE DENTISTRY
A PRACTICAL GUIDE

PATRICIA PENCE, DVM

Diplomat American Board of Veterinary Practitioners
Kimberly, Idaho

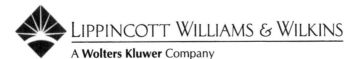

LIPPINCOTT WILLIAMS & WILKINS
A **Wolters Kluwer** Company

Philadelphia · Baltimore · New York · London
Buenos Aires · Hong Kong · Sydney · Tokyo

Editor: David Troy
Managing Editor: Dana Battaglia
Marketing Manager: Christine Kushner
Production Editor: Jennifer Ajello
Designer: Armen Kojoyian
Compositor: Maryland Composition
Printer: R.R. Donnelley & Sons-Crawfordsville
Cover Designer and Interior Designer: Karen Quigley

Library of Congress Cataloging-in-Publication Data

Pence, Patricia.
  Equine dentistry : a practical guide / Patricia Pence
    p. ; cm.
  Includes bibliographical references and index.
  ISBN 0-683-30403-8 (alk. paper)
  1. Horses—Diseases. 2. Veterinary dentistry. I. Title.
  [DNLM: 1. Tooth Diseases—veterinary. 2. Horse Diseases. 3. Mouth
Diseases—veterinary. SF 867 P397e 2002]
SF959.M66 P46 2002
636.1'08976—dc21

                                    2001050306

To purchase additional copies of this book, call our customer service department at **(800) 638-3030** or fax orders to **(301) 824-7390**. International customers should call **(301) 714-2324**.

Visit Lippincott Williams & Wilkins on the Internet: http://www.LWW.com. Lippincott Williams & Wilkins customer service representatives are available from 8:30 am to 6:00 pm, EST.

01 02 03 04 05
1 2 3 4 5 6 7 8 9 10

To the horses who have been our workmates, companions,
and friends through the centuries.

To the humans that recognize the suffering of this noble animal
and devote their lives to relieving that suffering.

To my mother, Bernice Pence, may she rest in peace,
and to Russ for instilling in me the attitude
that I can accomplish anything that I set my mind to.

PREFACE AND ACKNOWLEDGMENTS

In the overall scheme of things, I am a Johnny-Come-Lately to equine dentistry. In 1993 I bought a small animal and equine practice in Meridian, Idaho. My equine clientele was somewhat sparse at first, so I could devote plenty of time to my examinations. I had floated horses' teeth before, with the traditional long-straight and long-angled floats. Usually they had dull carbide chip blades on them because I didn't know when they were supposed to be changed. Now that I owned my own clinic, the quality of work I produced mattered more than ever. Even without a full-mouth speculum, I could see that floating was not going to correct some of the abnormalities that I could see in the anterior part of the oral cavity.

In the same year I received a catalogue in the mail from World Wide Equine, then located in Nebraska. I read about the equine dentistry school and longed to go. However, my cash flow at that time couldn't support the tuition, airfare, hotel, and loss of a week's wages. What really caught my eye was the Dremel-powered dental instruments in the catalogue. I thought about purchasing them, but decided against it. I intuitively realized that an untrained person could do much damage with equipment like that.

It wasn't until 1995 that I purchased a battery-operated Makita reciprocating float. I was sure this was going to be an excellent compromise, but after awhile, I discovered that it was just an improvement over what I had been doing. I floated many horses' teeth with that machine. I did not consider it to be an instrument. I wore it out in about 9 months and had a friend rebuild it.

In March of 1996, I heard that Dale Jeffrey and World Wide Equine had moved to my neck of the woods in Idaho. I also heard that there was some grumbling among the local veterinarians about a non-veterinarian practicing dentistry. There were no veterinarians to my knowledge practicing that type of advanced equine dentistry in the entire state at that time. (My apologies to those that were, if you are out there.) My curiosity and interest in dentistry got the best of me, so I visited him at his new place of business in Glenns Ferry, Idaho. Dale gave me the grand tour of his facilities—the School for Equine Dentistry, the instrument manufacturing company, and the showroom of dental equipment. I admired his collection of 100-plus horse skulls and listened with interest to theories about how certain abnormalities are generated. I asked him if he would come to my clinic and give me a private lesson on the use of the Dremel-operated instruments and the various floats. He complied graciously. During that lesson, he informed me that he was going to the University of California at Davis, Veterinary School to participate in a weekend equine dentistry workshop for California graduate veterinarians. As soon as he left, I called and registered for the course and bought a plane ticket to Sacramento. After that weekend, I became, as one Idaho veterinarian called me, a horse dentistry evangelist. I have been preaching to anyone within earshot ever since.

Armed only with the 2 hours of instruction that Dale Jeffrey gave me plus the weekend at Davis, I purchased about $500 worth of power instrumentation and floats from Dale. I was the classic example of someone who knew "just enough to be dangerous." But I proceeded cautiously and erred on the side of being conservative. I had to re-do a few horses, but as far as I know, I didn't ruin the mouths of any. Ignorance is bliss.

I was disappointed in the lack of printed information on equine dentistry. I had written three chapters for an avian textbook, Diseases of Cage and Aviary Birds, for the editors, Drs. Rosskopff and Woerpel 6 years before, so I was no stranger to accepting difficult writing projects on subjects in which I was not an expert. I called Carroll Cann, the managing editor for the avian book at Williams & Wilkins and asked if he was interested in publishing a textbook on equine dentistry. Carroll liked the table of contents I submitted and encouraged me to go for it.

I had no intention of writing the whole book. I merely wanted to write a couple of simple chapters and engage experts in the field to write the more technical chapters. I eventually found out how naïve I was, both about the magnitude of the project and my lack of appeal as an editor with no credentials. Fortunately, Kristin Wilewski found my enterprising spirit and enthusiasm appealing. Without her agreeing to write four of the technical chapters, I never would have proceeded. She and I share the same attitude toward life: "Jump, and a net will appear," is the way she describes it. I am indebted to Kristin for dropping nearly everything to write those chapters. Two years later I revised and expanded her chapters using what she had given me as the framework.

The #*&@! book project as it came to be called, had many false starts and many hiatus periods. Lippincott-Raven merged with Williams & Wilkins. Editors came and went. One editor, Dana Battaglia, stayed. A year ago I was despondent about how little I had accomplished in the previous 2 years and begged her to let me out of my contract. She begged me to persist, saying that a practical guide was needed.

A practical guide is what I offer to the student of equine dentistry. I am aware that I referenced too little and that I have omitted or avoided areas in which others may consider vital. But I included practice tips and highlighted key points so that the important concepts would stand out. After the dust settles and criticisms and suggestions are collected, I'll take what I've learned and make the next edition an even more practical guide to equine dentistry.

Many thanks to the above mentioned people. I would also like to thank the following equine dental technicians for their guidance in my own learning and for providing invaluable information regarding technique for the book: Tony Basile, Lance and Steve Rubin, Larry Moriarity, and Carl Mitz.

Thanks also to the following veterinarians: Gordon Baker, for reviewing the paper I submitted (on the surgical removal of a horizontally impacted PM2) as part of my American Board of Veterinary Practitioners application back in 1995, to Tom Allen for his kind remarks and encouraging words after reviewing one of the earliest versions of the book, to Richard Miller, Scott Greene, David Klugh, Randi Brannan, and Russ Tucker for reviewing chapters and providing suggestions. Thanks to Dale Jeffrey, Clay Stubbs, Harold Conrad, and Dennis Rach for providing photographs of instruments. Thanks also to Kevin May, Paulo Zaluski, Lloyd Jeffrey, and Lynn Caldwell just because you are nice to have around.

I'm sure I omitted someone who deserved my thanks. I hope to thank you later in person.

CONTRIBUTORS

PATRICIA PENCE, DVM

Diplomat American Board of Veterinary Practitioners
Kimberly, Idaho

KRISTEN WILEWSKI, DVM

International Association of Equine Dentists/Examiner
Poplar Grove, Illinois

TONY BASILE

Master Equine Dental Technician
International Association of Equine Dentists/Examiner
St. Helens, Oregon

SCOTT GREENE, DVM

International Association of Equine Dentists/Certified Advanced
Sparks, Nevada

CARL MITZ

Equine Dental Technician
International Association of Equine Dentists/Certified
Brenham, Texas

CONTENTS

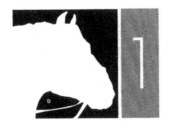

DENTAL ANATOMY

PATRICIA PENCE

The dentition of the horse is characterized by hypsodont teeth. Long crowns; short, late-forming roots; and no identifiable crown-root junction are defining features. Eruption is prolonged and facilitated with deposition of bone at the bottom of the alveolar socket as attrition occurs at the occlusal surface Bone 1. In comparison, humans, carnivores, and swine have brachydont teeth. The brachydont tooth is characterized by a distinctive crown, neck, and root. Enamel is restricted to the crown, and the tooth discontinues growing when the tooth is fully erupted.

Knowledge of the anatomy of normal dental and associated structures is necessary for the dental practitioner to be able to recognize, diagnose, and treat dental disease. An educated eye is needed to be able to identify pathology in individual teeth, whether that be identifying a supernumerary tooth, identifying a tooth with abnormal conformation, or differentiating caries from nonpathological discoloring. Imaging modalities used to differentiate between dental and nondental disease, i.e., radiology, computed tomography, magnetic resonance, and ultrasonography, depend heavily on a working knowledge of anatomy. For dental disease that requires surgical treatment, awareness of important structures that are in close apposition to the teeth is vital so that those structures may be protected from damage.

Understanding dental physiology is needed to appreciate how heavily mastication depends on normal anatomy. The practical implications of both anatomy and physiology are these: abnormalities in the height, shape, or composition of individual teeth can have profoundly negative effects on the dental system as a whole, as will be illustrated in later chapters.

This chapter will introduce the following basic concepts important to the understanding of normal anatomy of the equine dental system: the evolution of the dental system of the horse, embryology and development, nomenclature, and the

1

gross and applied anatomy of dental and associated structures. The chapter also describes the physiology of the dental system as it applies to mastication.

■ ■ EVOLUTION OF THE EQUINE DENTAL SYSTEM

The equine head and teeth illustrate the response of a species to evolutionary demands. The first known ancestor of the horse, Hyracotherium (also known as Eohippus), lived during the Lower Eocene period in South America.[1,2] It was a fox-sized creature that looked more like a small, hornless antelope than a modern horse. The face of this tiny creature was short, and the large eyes were set near the middle of the head. This primitive relative of the horse lived in jungles and forests and ate the soft, succulent vegetation that proliferated in the tropical climate of that period. The cheek teeth were smaller and simpler than those of modern equids.

After the Middle Miocene period, the environment and the diet of this creature changed. The earth's climate became cooler and dryer. The succulent, leafy plants were replaced by coarse, hardy grasses containing a high silica content. The teeth of the surviving descendants of Hyracotherium evolved to withstand the constant wear they were subjected to by a diet of abrasive grasses; such evolution allowed the animal to live long enough to maintain itself through the reproductive years. The skull became longer and deeper to accommodate the taller tooth crowns and larger teeth. The premolars became more complex and eventually became molars, creating a continuous grinding surface from the first to the last cheek tooth of each arcade.[1,2] Composed of elaborate patterns of cementum and dentin vertically folded with enamel, the cheek teeth became a lifelong supply of crown anchored by small roots. This folding created a self-sharpening grinding surface on the occlusal aspects of the cheek teeth and formed exaggerated sulci on the buccal surfaces of the maxillary teeth. Delayed maturation of the roots allowed the reserve crown to continue to grow after the exposed crown came into wear.

Another significant change was the development of an organ, the cecum, in which intestinal microbes digested plant material high in cellulose. Such coarse plant material needed to be ground into smaller particles for the horse than for ungulate species because the horse could not eructate its food back into the oral cavity for further chewing.

Approximately 5000 years ago, man domesticated the horse, changing its environment and diet considerably.[3] As human's environment changed from free-roaming and pastoral to agrarian and now, in many parts of the world, to urban, so did the environment and, more important, the diet of human's workmate and companion, the horse.

Horses kept in pens or stalls are fed twice a day and may spend only 4 hours a day grinding food, compared to the 16 or more hours a day that a pastured horse may spend grazing. The high silica plains grasses have been replaced by tender pasture grasses that are not as abrasive. Hay, hay cubes, and pelleted feed are picked up by the lips and by-pass working the incisors completely. The resulting lack of normal wear allows overgrowth of the incisors. Grain and pelleted feeds require shorter lateral–medial masticatory movements, thereby preventing use of the total molar grinding surfaces.[4] These unworn surfaces become sharp, overhanging edges on the buccal sides of the maxillary teeth and the lingual sides of the mandibular teeth.

■ ■ DEVELOPMENTAL ANATOMY

The embryonic mouth forms from an indentation of the ventral surface of the embryo at the level of the first branchial arch. An identifiable mouth cavity is present by the first 3 weeks in most species. At approximately 3½ weeks of age, a horseshoe-shaped band of cells appears composed of the ectodermal epithelium that lines the mouth. This band of cells forms two ridges, the vestibular lamina and the dental lamina. The vestibular lamina gives rise to the lips and gingiva. The dental laminae invaginate at predetermined intervals to create the first tissue of tooth formation, the enamel organ.[5–9]

The early development of hypsodont teeth is similar to branchydont teeth.[8,10] The enamel organ develops through a series of stages, differentiated by the shape of the enamel organ and the type of cells composing it. The initial invaginations of dental laminae, composed of ectoderm, mark the bud stage of the enamel organ. Deciduous tooth buds form first. Shortly thereafter, permanent tooth buds arise from the tissue that form the deciduous buds. During the next stage, the cap stage, the bud grows and forms a slight concavity. At this time, the enamel organ has three layers, all still ectoderm in origin. The enamel concavity deepens as the third, or bell stage, is entered. From this point on, the shape of the enamel organ depends on the type of tooth it is destined to become.

The individual layers of tooth tissue form during the bell stage. The cell layer lining the inside of the bell differentiates into ameloblasts at the apex and cementoblasts at the base. Eventually, the ameloblasts form the enamel layers, and the cementoblasts form the layers of cementum. The cells adjacent to the base of the bell originate from mesenchymal epithelial cells. These mesenchymal cells will align themselves against the epithelial cells lining the bell and differentiate into odontoblasts, which will form the dentin and pulp layers of the tooth. The odontoblasts and pulp are collectively called the dental papilla.

The enamel organ of hypsodont cheek teeth folds into a series of longitudinal cylinders that continue to grow distally *(Fig. 1.1)*.[10,11]When the tooth reaches its maximum length, the enamel organ covering the more mature, mineralized apical portion of the tooth degenerates. Distally, it continues to grow into the dental sac.

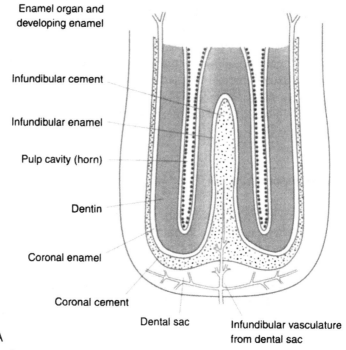

Enamel organ and
developing enamel

Infundibular cement

Infundibular enamel

Pulp cavity (horn)

Dentin

Coronal enamel

Coronal cement

Dental sac

Infundibular vasculature
from dental sac

A

Figure 1.1 The crown and occlusal surface of a multicusped hyposodont tooth with an infundibulum (i.e., an upper cheek tooth). A. Immediately prior to eruption. B. Immediately following eruption, showing loss of the dental sac over the occlusal surface. C. Following wear of the primary occlusal surface to expose the secondary occlusal surface that is the permanent occlusal surface in hyposodont teeth. (Reprinted with permission from: Baker GJ, Easley J. Equine Dentistry. Philadelphia: WB Saunders, 1999.)

The entire dental sac surrounding the hypsodont tooth differentiates into cementoblast cells, whereas only the layer of cells adjacent to the forming root become cementoblasts in the brachydont tooth. This complex will form a deciduous tooth.[11]

Deciduous teeth play an important role in dental development.[12] They act as guides for the proper placement of the permanent teeth. Therefore, their premature loss or delayed expulsion can cause maleruption or impaction of the permanent teeth. Permanent incisor and premolar teeth arise from the tissue of deciduous teeth. If the deciduous tooth bud does not form, no tooth will grow in its place.

Except for molars (teeth #9, 10, and 11), permanent teeth form from tissues of the deciduous teeth. The follicles of the developing permanent incisors lie lingual to the deciduous roots. The permanent premolar follicles lie within the bifurcation of the deciduous premolar roots.[10] The 12 molar teeth have no deciduous counterpart and branch directly off the dental lamina.[11] Pressure by the crown of the permanent tooth on the root of the decidous tooth causes resorption of the deciduous root. Re-

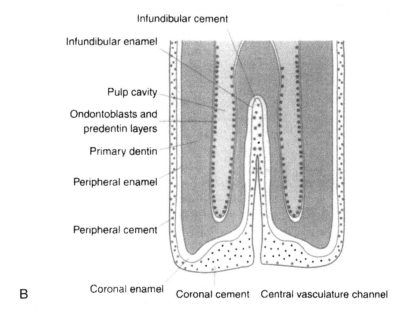

Infundibular cement

Infundibular enamel

Pulp cavity

Ondontoblasts and predentin layers

Primary dentin

Peripheral enamel

Peripheral cement

Coronal enamel   Coronal cement   Central vasculature channel

B

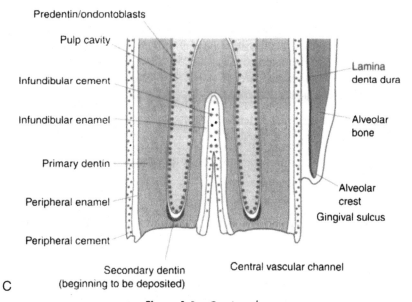

Predentin/ondontoblasts

Pulp cavity

Infundibular cement

Infundibular enamel

Primary dentin

Peripheral enamel

Peripheral cement

Lamina denta dura

Alveolar bone

Alveolar crest

Gingival sulcus

Secondary dentin (beginning to be deposited)   Central vascular channel

C

Figure 1.1 *Continued.*

TABLE 1.1   Eruption Schedule

	Tooth	0–1 year	1 year	2 years	3 years	4 years
Incisors	D #1	1st week				
	#1			2 years, 6 months		
	D #2	2 months				
	#2				3 years, 6 months	
	D #3	8 months				
	#3					4 years, 6 months
Canines	#4					4 years to 4 years, 6 months
Wolf Teeth	#5	6 months to 1 year				
Premolars	D #6	1st week				
	#6			2 years, 8 months		
	D #7	1st week				
	#7			2 years, 10 months		
	D #8	1st week				
	#8				3 years, 8 months	
Molars	#9		1 year			
	#10					
	#11			2 years		4 years

D = deciduous teeth
Note: This table serves as a guideline only. Some variation occurs between breeds.

sorption begins at the apical extremity of the tooth and continues in the direction of the crown until resorption of the entire root has taken place. The crown, which then loses its attachment owing to lack of support, is exfoliated during mastication.

Between the ages of 2½ years and 5 years, the dentition of the young horse is in a dynamic state. Twenty-four deciduous teeth will be shed, and 40 permanent teeth will erupt (*Table 1.1*).

> **KEY POINT**
> ▶ Premature loss or injury to deciduous teeth may cause permanent teeth to erupt in abnormal positions, be abnormally shaped, or fail to erupt at all.

■ ■ NOMENCLATURE

Dental Formulae

The denomination and number of teeth are described by the dental formula. Each tooth is represented by its first initial, I for incisor, C for canine, P for premolar, and M for molar, followed by the number of each type of tooth. The number of maxillary teeth is placed on a line above the number of mandibular teeth. The numbers of both are totaled, giving the number of teeth on one side of the mouth. Logically, doubling this number will give the total number of teeth. There are separate dental formalae for the deciduous teeth and the permanent teeth.

The **deciduous dental formula** for the horse is (I3/3 P3/3) × 2 = 24.

The **permanent dental formula** for the individual horse is variable, (I3/3 C1/1 P3 or 4/3 M3/3) × 2 = 40 to 44, depending on whether canine teeth and wolf teeth are present.

Tooth Surfaces

The surfaces[12] of the incisors and canines facing the lips are called the labial surfaces *(Fig. 1.2A, B).*

The surfaces of the cheek teeth in contact with the mucous membranes of skin overlying them are called the buccal surfaces. The tooth surfaces in contact with the tongue are called the lingual surfaces. The surfaces of the premolars and molars that contact those of the opposite jaw during the act of closure are called occlusal surfaces. In incisors, these contact surfaces are called incisal surfaces. The coronal portion of a tooth is the exposed crown. The reserve crown is the portion of the crown that is unexposed, i.e., below the gingival margin. The apical portion of a tooth is toward its root. This term is used to describe the reserve crown. The marginal border of a tooth is at the tooth–gingival interface.

The median line is drawn vertically between the central incisors at their point of contact with each other in both the maxilla and the mandible. The surfaces of teeth

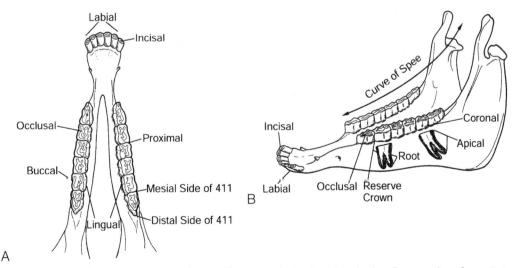

Figure 1.2   A. Dorsal view of the mandibular dental arch identifying tooth surfaces. **B.** Lateral view of the mandible, identifying tooth surfaces.

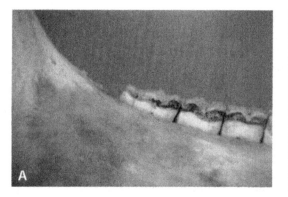

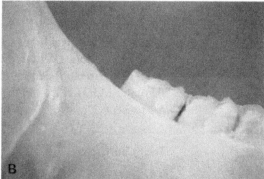

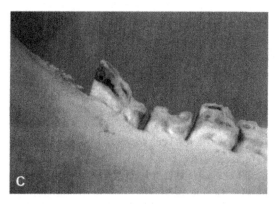

Figure 1.3 Lateral views of mandible showing normal and abnormal M3 (#11). **A.** This #11 tooth does not have a caudal hook and is placed somewhat low in the curve of spee. **B.** This #11 tooth is somewhat high in the curve of spee and could be mistaken for a hook. **C.** The caudal aspect of this #11 tooth is longer than the cranial aspect this is a true hook.

facing toward adjoining teeth in the same dental arch are called proximal surfaces. The proximal surfaces can be either mesial, the surface closest to or facing the median line, or distal, the surface farthest or facing away from the median line. The mesial surfaces of the cheek teeth are also referred to as rostral surfaces.

The curve of Spee is the anatomic curvature of the mandibular occlusal plane, beginning at the rostral surface of the second premolars (#06), following the buccal edges of the cheek teeth, and continuing to the anterior ramus of the mandible *(Fig. 1.3A–C)*. Knowledge of the existence of the curve of Spee becomes important when trying to differentiate between malocclusive and normal conditions of the last lower molars.

Numbering Systems

Numbering systems are used to identify individual teeth for record-keeping purposes. Currently, there are three numbering systems: the standard system, the cheek teeth system, and the modified Triadan system.

Standard System. The standard system is the one most familiar to veterinarians and students of anatomy. Each type of tooth is identified by the upper case letter assigned to it in the dental formula followed by a number assigning its position in the mouth relative to the median line *(Fig. 1.4A, B)*. Beginning with the incisors, the center incisors are called I1, the second incisors from the center are called I2, and the corner incisors I3. The first premolar, the wolf tooth, is called PM1, and the first cheek tooth is called PM2, etc. The drawback to this system is that confusion still exists about which specific tooth is being referred to unless it is separately specified whether the tooth is in the mandibular jaw or maxillary jaw, and on the right or left side.

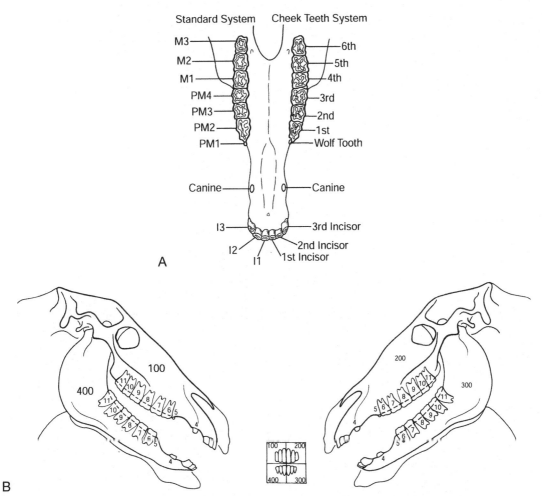

Figure 1.4   A. The standard and cheek teeth numbering systems. **B.** The Triadan numbering system is based on a full phenotypic dentition of 44 teeth. The teeth are numbered by quadrant and by tooth position. Upper right (quadrant 1), upper left (quadrant 2), lower left (quadrant 3), lower right (quadrant 4). Tooth position starts with numbering the central incisors #1. The canines are #4, the wolf teeth are #5, the first cheek teeth are #6, and the last cheek teeth are #11.

Cheek Teeth System. The cheek teeth system is similar to the standard system in that the incisors are numbered the same. However, the premolars and molars are referred to by number only, and the wolf teeth are not included as cheek teeth. The second premolar is called number one, the third premolar is called number two, and so on, ending with number six, the third molar *(Fig. 1.4A)*. A separate description must be added to identify whether the tooth is maxillary or mandibular, right or left.

Modified Triadan System. A third system, the modified Triadan numbering system, is becoming a more universal system of classifying individual teeth *(Fig. 1.4B)*.[13] This system divides the mouth into quadrants, to specify whether an individual tooth is in the upper or lower jaw and whether it is on the right or left side.

Moving clockwise, the right maxilla is called quadrant number one, and the teeth are labeled in the 100 series. Next the left maxilla is called quadrant number two, and the teeth are in the 200 series. Then follows the left mandible, called quadrant number three, and the teeth are in the 300 series; and the right mandible is called quadrant number four, and the teeth are in the 400 series. The teeth are then assigned another number according to their position relative to the median line, starting with the central incisor in that quadrant. Therefore, the first incisor is number one, the canine is number four, the wolf tooth is number five, and the last molar is number eleven.

■ ■   ANATOMY

Anatomically, the dental mechanism is designed to promote structural integrity and thereby prolong its own life. This structural integrity is maintained by the length and shape of the reserve crown, the angle at which occlusal surfaces are placed relative to the reserve crown and roots, adequate tooth substance for strength, and a biomechanical design that produces solidity with resistance against lines of force. The impressive mass of reserve crown relative to exposed crown anchors the tooth securely within its socket.[11] Although the incisors and cheek teeth are separated by the interdental space, each tooth within its group lies in close apposition to its neighbor. This tight arrangement helps stabilize the dental arches by the combined anchorage of all the teeth within each group and prevents food from lodging between the teeth and damaging the periodontium. The corner teeth, i.e., the third incisors (1/3, 2/3), the second premolars (1, 2, 3, 4/6), and the third molars (1, 2, 3, 4/11), are protected from drifting by the angle of direction of occlusal forces being in their favor and by the angulation of their occlusal surfaces with their roots.

Composition of Equine Teeth

Dentin. Equine teeth are composed primarily of dentin, a cream-colored substance composed of calcified tissue secreted by odontoblasts. The odontoblasts have their cell bodies in the pulp tissue and have long cytoplasmic processes that extend into the mineralized dentin tubules.[14] Approximately 70% of this tissue is mineral, primarily hydroxyapatite crystals. The remaining 30% is composed of collagen proteins, mucopolysaccharides, and water. The organic components give dentin the properties of elasticity and compressibility, which, as mentioned, helps protect the more brittle enamel components of equine teeth.

There are four types of dentin.[4] Primary dentin is produced during tooth development. Secondary dentin is deposited on the walls of the pulp canal and in the cytoplasmic processes. Tertiary dentin is produced to keep the pulp from being exposed as the occlusal surface is worn or as the result of an injury. Sclerotic dentin is produced in response to mild irritation.

KEY POINT
▶ Dentin protects the pulp from bacterial invasion as the pulp canal is exposed by wear.

Cementum. Cementoblasts produce cementum. Cementum covers the entire external surface of the tooth prior to eruption and fills the infundibuli of maxillary teeth and incisors. Similar to dentin in composition, cementum is approximately 65% mineral, 35% organic material, and water.[15] Supragingival cementum has no blood supply after eruption and serves to fill in surface irregularities and to protect the enamel. Subgingival cementum is part of the peridontal ligament complex and is living tissue. Cementoblasts in the alveolus secrete cementum in response to tooth eruption and to infection or injury.

Enamel. Enamel is the hardest substance in the body. Secreted by ameloblasts, enamel is approximately 98% hydroxyapatite crystals and 2% keratinous proteins. Enamel is an inert substance, not a living tissue, and therefore cannot reproduce or repair itself. The high mineral content of enamel gives this substance high tensile strength but also makes it brittle. Supporting layers of dentin and cementum absorb the shock applied to teeth and prevent the enamel from chipping and cracking. This layering of dental substances protects the enamel and enables the exposed edges to act as self-sharpening blades to shred roughage.

Electron microscopic examination of sections of teeth has shown equine enamel to have different structures depending on where in the tooth it is laid down.[16] Three types of equine enamel have been described and classified according to the structure and arrangement of the hydroxyapatite crystals.

KEY POINT
▶ The brittle enamel layer is protected from shattering by support from the more elastic dentin and cementum layers.

Pulp. Pulp is a loose connective tissue composed of arteries, veins, nerves, lymphatics, odontoblasts, and fibroblasts that occupies the pulp cavity of the tooth.[4] Its primary function is to support and nourish the dentin-producing odontoblasts. Pulp's extensive nerve supply gives the tooth sensory capabilities, thereby giving the tooth defensive capabilities. When irritation is detected, the odontoblasts respond by secreting dentin to protect the injured area.[12]

Incisors. The incisors of horses are used to nip and tear off forage and for defense. Incisors have a single enamel-lined infundibulum that presents at eruption as a cup in the incisal surface. As the tooth is worn down, the infundibum tapers to a white spot of enamel that is lost to attrition when the horse is approximately 15 years old *(Fig 1.5).*[17]

The roots of incisors contain a single pulp canal and terminate in a single apex. The pulp canal fills with secondary dentin when wear or injury exposes it.

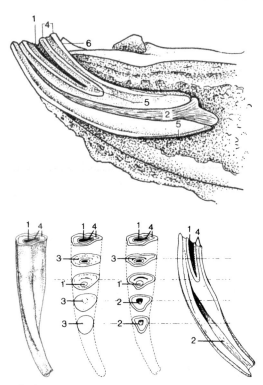

Figure 1.5 Structure of a lower incisor. *A, In situ,* sectioned longitudinally; the clinical crown is short in relation to the embedded part of the tooth. *B,* Caudal view; the junction between the clinical crown and the rest of the tooth is not marked. *C,* As a result of wear the occlusal surface changes; the cup gets smaller and disappears, leaving, for a time, the enamel spot; the dental star appears and changes from a line to a large round spot. *D,* These are sawn sections of a young tooth for comparison. *E,* longitudinal section of incisor, showing the relationship between the infundibulum and dental cavity; the latter is rostral.

The shape of the incisal surface and the exposed crown changes from oval, to round, then finally triangular as attrition occurs.[18] The angle of eruption also changes with age and wear because the curve of the reserve crown is flatter than the crown initially erupted. The incisors of the young horse erupt in an almost vertical fashion. As the horse matures, the angle diverges more toward the horizontal.

The upper corner incisors may have a vertical groove in the center of the labial surface. This landmark, known as Galvayne's groove, appears at approximately age 10, extends the length of the tooth at approximately age 20, will be half gone sometime near age 25, and will be completely gone by approximately age 30.[16,19] This groove is not always present and can be hard to see unless it is discolored.

Distinct differences between the deciduous and permanent incisors exist that assist aging the horse by incisor eruption and wear. Deciduous teeth are smaller and whiter, have a constricted neck, and are well-worn. Deciduous teeth do not have an infundibulum. Permanent teeth are larger, are covered by yellowish cementum, have no identifiable neck, and have distinct vertical ridges.

KEY POINT
▶ Anatomical landmarks on incisors have been used for centuries to estimate the age of horses.[19]

Canine teeth. Canine teeth are used for fighting and are usually found only in male horses. Male horses usually have one canine tooth per arcade in the large interdental space between the incisors and molars. Sometimes one or more are missing, or rarely, there is more than one in an arcade. Occasionally, female horses erupt canine teeth, but they are usually only in the mandible and are very small *(Fig. 1.6)*. Canine teeth have a large root that comprises ⅔ to ¾ the length of the tooth.

It is common for canine teeth to be thickly coated with tartar, which can cause mild-to-moderate periodontal disease at the gingival margin.

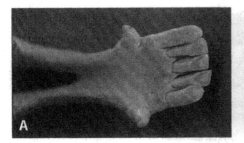 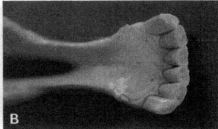

Figure 1.6 **A.** Canine teeth in a mature male horse. **B.** Canine teeth in a mature female horse.

Wolf teeth. The first premolar, commonly called the wolf tooth, is a small, rudimentary tooth. Usually present in both sides of the maxillary arcade in close proximity to the first cheek teeth, these teeth have distinct necks and roots. Wolf teeth may be found more cranially in the interdental space, may be found in the mandibular arcade, there may be more than one per quadrant, they may present as unerupted teeth, and they may be completely absent. Wolf teeth also vary in size of crown and root and, not surprisingly, ease of extraction.

KEY POINT

▶ The palatine artery lies in close proximity (2 to 3 mm medial) to the lingual gingival margin of the maxillary teeth and must be avoided when teeth are extracted.

Cheek teeth. The cheek teeth are designed to be continuously erupting, self-sharpening grinders. This self-sharpening is facilitated by the presence of enamel-lined infundibuli in the maxillary arcades *(Fig. 1.7)*. A layer of cementum fills the infundibulum and folds with layers of enamel and dentin to form lophs. These

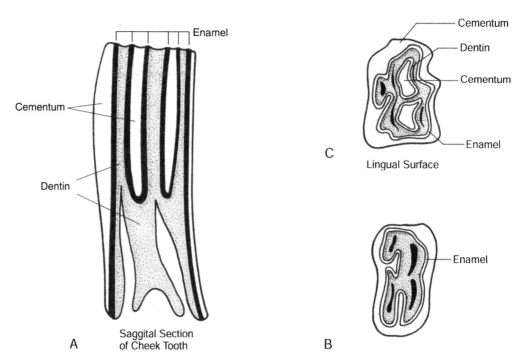

Figure 1.7   A. Sagittal section of molar. **B.** Occlusal surface of maxillary tooth. **C.** Occlusal surface of mandibular tooth.

different dental substances wear at different rates, resulting in an irregular occlusal surface.

KEY POINT

▶ The occlusal surface wears away at a rate of 2 to 3 mm per year.[20] The horse's diet and the presence of sand in the food may alter this rate.

The 12 decidous premolars (#6, 7, and 8) are erupted at birth or within the first week. These temporary teeth shed at approximately 2 years, 8 months; 2 years, 10 months; and 3 years, 8 months of age. The permanent molars (# 9, 10, and 11) erupt at approximately 1, 2, and 3.5 years of age.

The upper and lower cheek teeth have several distinct anatomical differences. Maxillary cheek teeth have two infundibuli, but the mandibular teeth have none. The maxillary teeth are more wide and square than the mandibular teeth and have pronounced longitudinal ridges on their buccal aspects. These enamel ridges can be very sharp on their ventral corners and are the source of a great deal of discomfort. The mandibular teeth are more narrow and oblong and do not have longitudinal ridges (*Fig. 1.8A,B*).

At eruption, the permanent cheek tooth consists of an exposed crown, a reserve crown with a widely dilated apex, and 5 or 6 pulp horns that connect to a pulp chamber in the reserve crown. Root walls are immature, consisting of just a thin plate of enamel.[21]

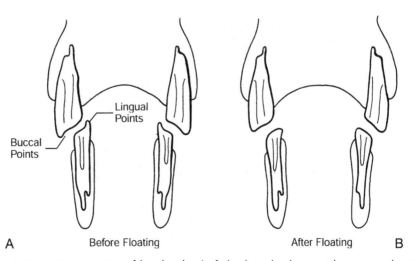

Figure 1.8 **A.** Cross section of head at level of cheek teeth, showing sharp enamel points. **B.** Cross section of head at level of cheek teeth, showing appearance after floating.

Two years after eruption, root walls are still thin and contain wide pulp canals that converge into a pulp chamber. Growth continues at the distal end of the permanent cheek tooth until approximately 7 years after eruption. During this period of tooth growth and maturation, it is typical to see swellings on the ventral aspect of the mandible. These swellings are most pronounced in 3-year-old and 4-year-old horses. Occasionally, the swellings do not disappear and are a permanent part of the ventral contour of the mandible. Unless there is drainage from the roots, they are not clinically significant.

Roots mature during a period of 6 to 8 years, during which they are strengthened by depositing dentin inside the root and cementum on the outside. The true roots of equine teeth are in the apical areas and contain no enamel.[22]

The endodontic system of the maturing cheek tooth consists of two roots in mandibular teeth (except for the 11's, which have three roots) and three (sometimes four) roots in maxillary teeth. The root canals lead to a shrinking common pulp chamber. Deposition of dentin causes the size of the pulp chamber to become smaller with age until it all but disappears at approximately 6 years' posteruption.

Supporting Structures

Teeth are supported within horseshoe-shaped bony ridges in the mandible and maxilla called the dental arches. Each dental arch is composed of a right and a left alveolar process.

The alveolar process contains several bony layers: the lamina dura, cortical bone, and trabecular bone *(Fig. 1.9)*. The lamina dura is the thin layer of bone that forms the wall of the alveolus; cortical bone forms the dense, supportive outer layer of bone. Trabecular bone is the spongy osseous tissue within the dense layers of cortical bone. The roots of the teeth are imbedded in osseous sockets, called alveoli, and

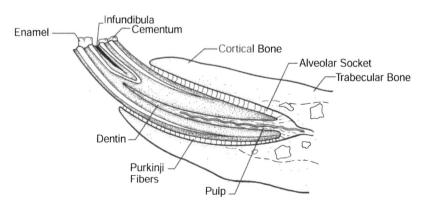

Figure 1.9 Sagitttal section of alveolar process of an incisor showing tooth, apical foramen, pulp, artery, vein, and nerve entering tooth, periodontal ligament, lamina dura, cortical bone, and trabecular bone.

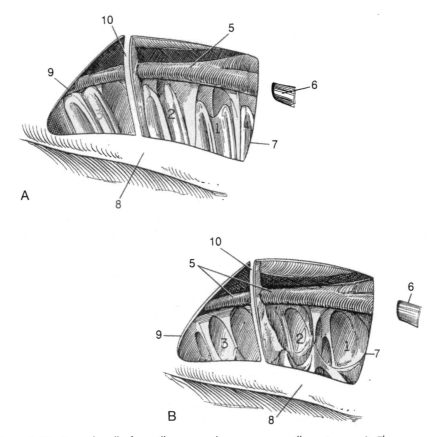

Figure 1.10 Lateral wall of maxilla removed to expose maxillary sinuses. **A**, Three years of age. **B**, Thirteen years of age. 1, 2, 3 = Alveoli covering roots of first, second, and third molars, respectively; 4 = alveolus covering root of fourth premolar; 5 = infraorbital canal; 6 = infraorbital nerve emerging from infraorbital canal; 7 = rostral maxillary sinus; 8 = facial crest; 9 = caudal maxillary sinus; 10 = septum.

are attached to bone by fibers in the periodontal ligament, called Sharpy's fibers. The periodontal ligament suspends and attaches the tooth to the lamina dura. Proprioceptive nerves in the periodontal ligament send messages to the brain about the position of the mandible.

Sinuses. The sinuses of most importance relative to dentistry in the horse are the rostral and caudal maxillary sinuses *(Fig. 1.10A)*. Owing to the length of the reserve crowns, the roots of the upper #8, #9, and #10 protrude into the rostral maxillary sinus (usually after the age of twelve, the roots of #8 no longer project into the sinus). The roots of upper #11 similarly protrude into the caudal maxillary sinuses.[23] By then, the reserve crown has, for the most part, been used up, leaving only the exposed crown and the roots. The roots are covered by a thin layer of bone, which is,

> **BOX 1.1   SURGICAL BOUNDARIES OF THE MAXILLARY SINUSES**
>
> Caudal: Rostral limit of the orbit.
> Rostral: A line connecting the end of the facial crest to the infraorbital canal.
> Ventral: The facial crest.
> Dorsal: A line from the infraorbital foramen parallel to the facial crest.

in effect, the floor of the sinus *(Fig. 1.10B)*. Damage to the tooth root by disease or injury can dissolve the bone overlying it, creating a communicating tract through which exudate can drain into the sinus, exiting through the nasomaxillary aperture and out the nostril. Although the rostral and caudal maxillary sinuses are separated by a septum, the dorsal aspect is thin and can be eroded by the enzymes in purulent exudates. Knowledge of the boundaries of the maxillary sinuses is necessary to create an appropriate window for surgery (*Box 1.1*).

The rostral maxillary sinus communicates with the ventral conchal sinus. The caudal maxillary sinus communicates with the sphenopalatine sinus, which in turn communicates with the conchofrontal sinus through the frontomaxillary opening.

Therefore, inflammation of any of these structures can lead to a nasal discharge, creating the need to differentiate sinus disease from dental disease in any horse young enough to have tooth roots intimately associated with sinus structures.

KEY POINT
> ▶ The infraorbital canal is closely associated with the roots of the upper 08 (caudal root), #9, #10, and, #11 cheek teeth. The nasolacrimal canal travels just beneath the surface of the maxilla, dorsal, and lateral to the infraorbital canal. Both of these structures may be injured by trauma and must be preserved during surgical treatment of disease in the upper cheek teeth (*Box 1.1*).

Muscles of Mastication (Fig. 1.11). The masseter muscle is the largest and strongest muscle in this group because of the tremendous force necessary to crush grain and mature plant stems. It originates superficially on the facial crest and deeply on the zygomatic arch. The masseter muscle has fibers that run both vertically and caudolaterally around the mandible. This anatomic arrangement facilitates lateral and rotational movements by the mandible, the only moveable bone in the skull. The medial and lateral pterygoideus muscles assist the masseter muscle in unilateral contractions and horizontal jaw movements. The medial pterygoideus is responsible for the powerful lingual stroke of the mastication cycle.[18]

The temporalis muscle originates on the temporal fossa and medial surface of the zygomatic arch. It inserts on the coronoid process of the mandible. The temporalis muscle elevates the mandible and presses it against the maxilla. The digastricus muscle and the mylohyoides muscle lie within the intermandibular space. The digastricus muscle opens the mouth, and the mylohyoideus muscle controls tongue movement.

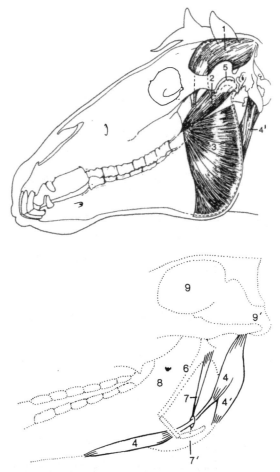

Figure 1.11 Drawings of skull, showing muscles of mastication. (Reprinted with permission from: Dyce KM, Sack WO, Wensing CJG. Textbook of Veterinary Anatomy. 2nd ed. Philadelphia: WB Saunders.)

KEY POINT

▶ Atrophy or hypertrophy of the temporalis or masseter muscles may be seen secondary to dental disease. Muscle atrophy will be present if the dental arcades on one side are not being used, and hypertrophy will be present on the side that is being used exclusively.

Temporomandibular joint. The temporomandibular joint of the horse is wider in medial–lateral articular surface area than that of carnivores or humans, allowing greater side-to-side gliding motion. The joint also works in a loose hinge-like manner, allowing some anterior–posterior motion. The mandibular condyle forms a diarthrodial joint with the mandibular fossa of the temporal bone. The joint is surrounded externally by a joint capsule and is lined internally with synovial membrane. Synovial fluid and a central meniscus cushion the articular cartilage.

KEY POINT

▶ Dental abnormalities can apply abnormal pressure on one or both temporomandibular joints, causing pain and even degenerative joint disease.

Nerve supply to the teeth. The mandibular branch of the trigeminal nerve innervates the skin and oral mucous membranes. It also gives motor innervation to the muscles of mastication. The buccal nerve has both sensory and parasympathetic fibers. It supplies the oral mucous membranes and buccal salivary glands. The lingual nerve supplies sensory innervation to the rostral two-thirds of the tongue and has parasympathetic fibers to the sublingual and mandibular salivary glands.

The inferior alveolar nerve enters the mandibular canal on the medial surface of the mandible. Within the mandible, it sends branches to the mandibular teeth; then, it exits the mandible via the mental foramen.

The maxillary teeth are supplied by a large branch of the maxillary nerve, the infraorbital nerve. The infraorbital nerve enters the infraorbital canal and gives off branches to the teeth in the maxilla. It exits from the infraorbital foramen and branches to supply sensation to the upper lip, nostrils, and nasal vestibule. The infraorbital canal is closely associated with the roots of maxillary cheek teeth PM4 (#8), M1 (#9), M2 (#10), and M3 (#11).

KEY POINT

▶ Knowledge of the nerves that provide sensation to the teeth is useful when local anesthesia is desired prior to painful procedures.

Salivary glands. Saliva is a bicarbonate-rich fluid produced by exocrine cells in the various salivary glands. Saliva is important for predigestion of food by adding moisture and amylase, an enzyme needed for carbohydrate breakdown. The bicarbonate in saliva is also important for preserving systemic acid–base balance.

The major salivary glands in the horse are the parotid, the mandibular, the sublingual, and the buccal glands. The parotid is the largest salivary gland, extending from the base of the ear dorsally to the linguofacial vein ventrally and occupying the space behind the caudal border of the mandible. Saliva is collected in several smaller ducts and is transported to the mouth via the large parotid duct. The parotid duct associates with the facial artery and vein as they follow the ventral border of the mandible around to the lateral surface of the face. The duct opens into the mouth at the level of the second or third upper cheek tooth.[18]

The smaller mandibular gland lies beneath the parotid gland, the tendon of insertion of the sternomandibularis, the digastricus, and the maxillary vein. The mandibular duct associates with the mylohyoideus muscle and follows the sublin-

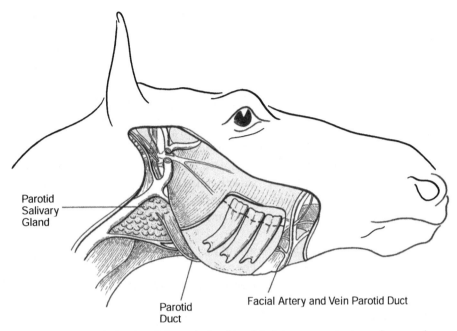

Figure 1.12 Parotid gland and duct relationship of facial artery and vein as they travel beneath the mandible.

gual gland, opening with it into the sublingual caruncle on the floor of the mouth just caudal to the incisors.

The sublingual gland is polystomatic in the horse. It lies directly beneath the oral mucosa between the tongue and the medial surface of the mandible from the third cheek tooth to the level of the chin. The sublingual gland has many small ducts that open on papillae below the tongue.

The buccal glands lie with the buccinator muscle in the cavity beneath the facial crest.

There are also microscopic salivary glands in the tongue, lips, and soft palate.

KEY POINT

▶ The parotid duct (and facial artery and vein) pass along the ventral edge of the mandible at the level of lower cheek teeth 10 and 11 and need to be preserved when surgical treatment of disease of these teeth is necessary (*Fig. 1.12*).

■ ■ DENTAL PHYSIOLOGY

For each species, the dental system has evolved to efficiently process the food substances most commonly available to it into a form that can be easily digested by its unique digestive system. The dental system of the horse was designed to crush and shred plant material high in cellulose into particles small enough for nutrients to be extracted by microbial fermentation. The teeth in one arcade engage into occlusion laterally; then, they slide at a medial–dorsal angle, shearing the fibers in roughage-based food. Next, the teeth are disengaged, allowing the mandible to rotate laterally in a dorsal arc, beginning a new cycle. The structure of hypsodont teeth coupled with rotational masticatory movements create self-sharpening, grinding surfaces that break and shred roughage into a bolus that travels from the rostral aspect of the oral cavity caudally to be swallowed.

The largest facial muscles in the horse are those used to close the mandible, the temporalis and masseter muscles. These muscles are bulky and overdeveloped compared to those of the carnivorous mammals and humans. The tremendous forces required to crush stems and grain are much greater than those needed to shear the soft tissues of meat.

The loph design of the cheek teeth create an ideal surface to shred roughage after it is crushed. The softer dentin and cementum substances wear first, allowing the exposed enamel portions of the loph to act as self-sharpening blades. The fissure between the enamel ridges of the lophs channel masticated feed material back into the center of the oral cavity. There, it is squeezed by the tongue against the paired and slightly offset palatine ridges to be extruded back onto a more caudal chewing sur-

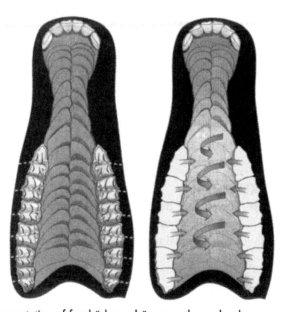

Figure 1.13 Representation of food "channels" across the occlusal surace of maxillary cheek teeth and their relationship to palatine ridges. (Reprinted with permission from: Baker GJ, Easley J. Equine Dentistry. Philadelphia: WB Saunders, 1999.)

face for further mastication. As the food bolus is rolled during mastication, it forms a spindle shape, which gives support to the theory of the rostral–caudal, auger–like action (*Fig. 1.13*).[24]

Finally, the grinding surfaces are continually replaced by the reserve crown of the hypsodont tooth until the tooth is worn down to its roots.

The dental apparatus of the horse was designed to work efficiently as long as the occlusal surfaces of each tooth are worn at the same rate as the rest of the teeth. However, owing to variations in tooth and jaw size, tooth composition, delayed or premature shedding of deciduous teeth, congenital defects, and trauma, individual horses rarely have ideal dentition.

■ ■ REFERENCES

1. Hope CEG, Jackson GN, eds. The Encyclopedia of the Horse. New York: The Viking Press,
2. Bennet D. The evolution of the horse. In: Evans JW, ed. Horse Breeding and Management. Amsterdam: Elsevier:1–29.
3. Edwards EH. The Encyclopedia of the Horse. New York: Dorling Kindersly Publishing, Inc., 1994.
4. Easley J. Equine dental development and anatomy. In: In-depth Dentistry Seminar, Proceedings of the American Association of Equine Practitioners, 1996. Vol. 42, pp. 1–10.
5. Noden DM, de Lahunta A. The Embryology of Domestic Animals: Developmental Mechanisms and Malformations. Baltimore: Williams & Wilkins,
6. Larsen WJ. Human Embryology. New York: Churchill Livingstone, 1993.
7. Warshawsky H. The teeth. In Weiss L, ed. Histology, 5th ed. New York: Macmillan Press, 1983:609–655.
8. Fortelius M. Ungulate cheek teeth: developmental, functional and evolutionary interrelations. Acta Zoologica Fennica 1984;18:1–76.
9. Ten Cate AR. Development of the tooth and its supporting tissues. In: Ten Cate AC, ed. Oral Histology, 4th ed. St. Louis: CV Mosby, 1994:58–80, 111–119, 147–168.
10. Misk NA, Sellem SM. Radiographic studies on the development of cheek teeth in donkeys. Equine Practice 1997;19(2):27–38.
11. Latshaw WK. Face, mouth, and pharynx. In: Latshaw WK, ed. Veterinary Developmental Anatomy—A Clinically Oriented Approach. Toronto: BC Decker Inc., 1987:95–100.
12. Wheeler RC. Dental Anatomy, Physiology, and Occlusion, 5th ed. Philadelphia: WB Saunders Company, 1974:25–47, 98–103, 405–504
13. Lowder MQ. Current nomenclature for the equine dental arcade. Vet Med 1998; Aug:753–755.
14. Kilic S, Dixon PM, Kempson SA. A light microscopic and ultrastructural examination of calcified dental tissues of horses. I: The occlusal surface and enamel thickness. Equine Veterinary Journal 1997;29:3, 190–197.
15. Kilic S, Dixon PM, Kempson SA. A microscopic light and ultrastructural examanination of calcified dental tissues of horses. II: Ultrastructural enamel findings. Equine Veterinary Journal 1997;29:198–205.

16. Kilic S, Dixon PM, Kempson SA. A light microscopic and ultrastructural examination of calcified dental tissues of horses. III: Dentine. Equine Veterinary Journal 1997;29:3, 206–212.

17. McMullen WC. Dental criteria for estimating age in the horse. Equine Practice 1983; 5, 10, 36.

18. Budras KD, Sack WO. Anatomy of the Horse: An Illustrated Text. London: Mosby-Wolfe, 1994.

19. Kertesz P. A Colour Atlas of Veterinary Dentistry & Oral Surgery. London: Wolfe, 1993.

20. Baker GJ. Oral examination and diagnosis: management of oral diseases. In: Veterinary Dentistry, Baker GJ and Easley J, eds. WB Saunders, Philadelphia 1999.

21. Kirkland KD, Baker GJ, Manfra-Marretta S, et al. Effects of aging on the endodontic system, reserve crown, and roots of equine mandibular cheek teeth. Am J Vet Res 1996;51(1):31.

22. De Lahunta A, Habel RE. Applied Veterinary Anatomy. Philadelphia: WB Saunders, 1986:4–16.

23. Hillman DJ. The skull. In: Getty R, ed. Sisson and Grossman's Anatomy of Domestic Animals. Vol. 1, 5th ed. Philadelphia: WB Saunders, 1975:499, 504.

24. Baker GJ. Dental physiology. In: Baker GJ, Easley J, eds. Equine Dentistry. Philadelphia: WB Saunders, 1999:29–34.

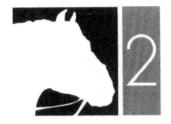

DENTAL EQUIPMENT

PATRICIA PENCE

The evolution of equipment designed specifically for equine dentistry progressed rapidly during the 1990s. Motorized and air-driven dental instruments and solid carbide float blades have made the practice of equine dentistry more professionally rewarding and less physically demanding. These improvements in working conditions plus training courses in advanced dentistry and an increase in documentation and exchange of information have contributed greatly to increased interest in equine dentistry. This chapter introduces modern dentistry instruments and associated equipment.

Although suppliers of some of some unique equipment will be mentioned in this, it is impossible to list the suppliers of each instrument. The reader is encouraged to order catalogs from all the dealers mentioned in Appendix A and to try out equipment at professional meetings and workshops.

■■ PROPER TECHNIQUE AND BODY POSTURE

No doubt, the new instruments have relieved dentists of much of the physical strength that was required when tools were limited. However, performing dentistry on horses is still demanding work. Improper technique and body posture causes unnecessary fatigue and even musculoskeletal injury.

Standing in a hunched position can cause lower back pain. If possible, stand with your back and shoulders straight and perpendicular to the ground *(Fig. 2.1)*. If you have to work at a slightly lower position, keep your back straight, and bend your knees. Spreading your legs wider will take some of the strain off your thighs. As long

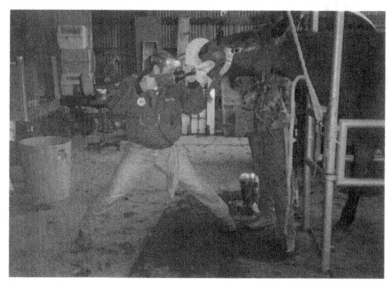

Figure 2.1   A widespread stance allows you to lower your body and keep your back straight without excessive strain on your thighs.

as you do not compromise your safety, use a stool to sit on if you have to work too low to squat just a little. Raise or lower the horse's head so you can work in a more comfortable position. Stand on a box if you are short or the horse is excessively tall so you do not strain to reach into its mouth.

PRACTICE TIP:

Using your dominant hand all the time can lead to crippling tendonitis or elbow arthritis. Repetitive motion injuries are common when one arm does all the work. Hand floating is the worst culprit for this. The solution, although admittedly not an easy one, is to learn to float with your nondominant hand. Start by doing routine tasks, like brushing your teeth, writing, or hammering nails into a board with your nondominant hand. It is frustrating and difficult at first, but just as anything else, it becomes easier the more you practice.

Modern dental instruments work most efficiently when they are sharp and when they are applied with just the right amount of pressure. Keep sharp float blades and burrs on your instruments, and you will get the job done faster. Let the instruments do the work. Sharp instruments work better if you just stroke them across the teeth. Grinding them into the teeth only creates more friction and is just wasted energy. If you must apply a considerable amount of pressure to get the job done, then your instruments are too dull.

■ ■ MISCELLANEOUS EQUIPMENT

A flat surface to lay out instruments, sedatives, syringes, etc., will make everything easier to find and keep them cleaner as well *(Fig. 2.2)*. In addition, it creates a more professional appearance. A portable camp table that rolls up for transport and storage is ideal. The table is easy to set up, clean up, and take apart. It is also inexpensive and can be found in most stores that carry camping supplies *(Box 2.1)*.

An adequate light source is essential to perform a thorough oral examination and to do the necessary dental work. Options include headlamps, flashlights, movable surgery lights, halogen work lights, or fiberoptic lights. Having more than one light source is often best; be sure to bring spare bulbs and batteries.

Long-handled mechanics mirrors and endoscopes can also help visualize the tooth surfaces difficult to see from the dentist's viewpoint, such as the spaces between teeth.

You will need a bucket of water with antiseptic in it in which to place your instruments. Some dentists put each float into a polyvinylchloride (PVC) pipe tube (Harlton Products and Olsen and Silk Abrasives), which clamps to the inside edge of the bucket, to keep their expensive solid carbide floats from scraping against one another *(Fig. 2.3)*. You will need a brush with stiff, nonrusting bristles to clean float heads, cut-off wheels, and Dremel burrs. A large-dose syringe to rinse the mouth out before, during, and after the dental procedure is also needed.

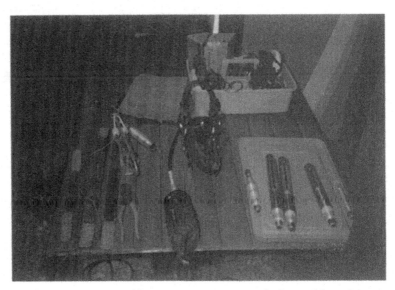

Figure 2.2 A roll-up camp table to put instruments on is both portable and inexpensive.

BOX 2.1   MISCELLANEOUS EQUIPMENT

Portable table
Light source
Extension cords
Multiplug power
Bucket
Antiseptic
Cleaning brush
Retractors
Extra-large halter and lead rope
Headstand
Dental halter
Ground fault breaker

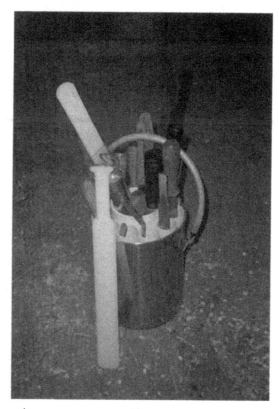

Figure 2.3 Bucket with instruments protected by PVC tubes. The flat, white paddles are used to displace and protect the tongue when using rotary instruments.

⸪ **PRACTICE TIP:**
Keep a large halter with your equipment because most of your clients' halters will not allow the jaws to open wide enough.

Soft-tissue retractors are valuable for pulling the commissure of the lips away from the teeth you are working on and for pushing the caudal part of the tongue out of the way. Retractors both improve visualization and help prevent damage to soft tissues. Equi-Dent makes a stainless steel buccal retractor that shields as well as retracts the buccal mucosa when burrs are being used. Malleable Army-Navy surgical retractors also perform as buccal retractors. When one more set of hands is needed and not available, bungee cords can be used as buccal retractors by slipping one hook into the commissure, pulling the cord snug, and hooking the other hook wherever you can. Retractors and tongue shields can be handmade by cutting up polyurethane cutting boards made for kitchen use.

Some means of supporting the head of the sedated horse is considered essential by most people who often perform dentistry out in the field. One way of accomplishing this is to use a portable headstand *(Fig. 2.4)*. The part of the stand that the mandibles rest on needs to be heavily padded and have a washable cover. The stand

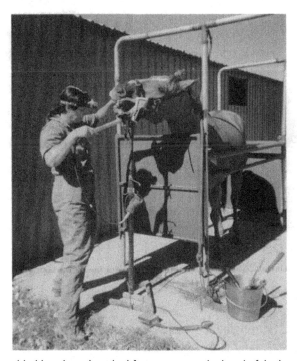

Figure 2.4. A padded headstand is ideal for supporting the head of the horse when performing dentistry out in the field.

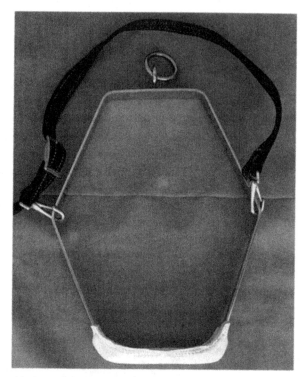

Figure 2.5   A padded metal dental halter can be used to suspend the horse's head in place of a headstand.

must be adjustable so that changes in height can be made quickly and easily. An alternative means of supporting the head during dental procedures is to use a dental halter *(Fig. 2.5)*. This is a special halter that has a rigid, oversized noseband. Because the noseband is rigid and is sprung away from the nose, there is enough room to use a speculum while still having plenty of clearance away from the cheeks. The head is suspended by a rope attached to the top of the noseband that is looped over a hook or ceiling beam. This allows the head to be quickly raised or lowered as needed. You can also suspend the head by attaching a rope to the noseband of the full-mouth speculum.

■ ■   **GAGS AND SPECULA**

Through the years, many types of specula have been developed for use on the horse *(Figs. 2.6, 2.7)*. Mouth gags hold the mouth open by being wedged between the cheek teeth, usually on just one side of the mouth. They are used when access to the cheek teeth on just one side is needed. Occasionally, they are used for incisor procedures.

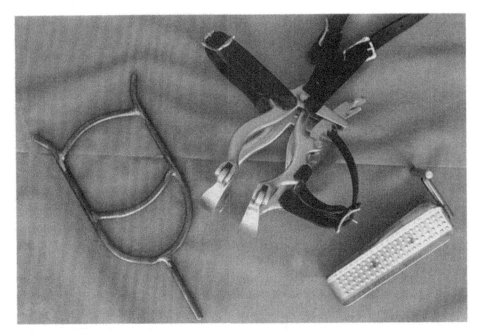

Figure 2.6 Clockwise from top: pig or bovine gag, full-mouth speculum, gag or wedge speculum.

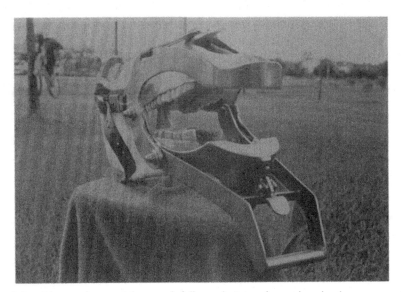

Figure 2.7 A heavy-duty, stainless-steel, full-mouth Conrad speculum that has convex side bars to prevent interference while working on the buccal edges of the upper cheek teeth. The ratchet mechanism is below the chin and out of the way of a headstand or dental halter.

The most common shapes of the bearing surface of the gags are wedge-shaped and spool-shaped. The wedge-shaped gags are by far the safer of the two because they distribute the pressure exerted by the jaws over the surfaces of several cheek teeth. Spool-shaped gags are not recommended because the pressure is concentrated on just one upper and lower tooth. If the horse chews hard on a spool speculum, a cheek tooth could be fractured or the gag could slip medially and cause injury to the palate. Because they are more flexible, wedge gags that use hard rubber or polyurethane as the wedge are more comfortable to the horse than unpadded stainless steel gags. Horses inevitably chew on the gags, and the temporomandibular joint on the unsupported side can be strained and cause pain.

Another type of gag speculum is one previously advertised as a pig or bovine gag. This is a simple piece of equipment used to pry open the mouth and keep it open by applying pressure on the upper and lower bars. The operator needs to use one hand or have the aid of an assistant to hold the speculum in place. Although obviously uncomfortable for the horse, these gags can be used to obtain brief glimpses at the cheek teeth to look for foreign bodies wedged in the mouth or to roughly estimate the cost of dentistry. They should not be used for dental procedures.

The full-mouth speculum is the most useful of the group. A full-mouth speculum is imperative to perform good dentistry on the cheek teeth. The full-mouth speculum fixes open the oral cavity so the practitioner can palpate and visualize individual teeth without interference by the speculum itself. When properly adjusted, there is equal pressure on both sides, which avoids temporomandibular strain during the procedure. Heavy sedation is required when using the full-mouth speculum to calm the horse and to encourage it to relax its jaw muscles and tongue.

Full-mouth specula are made for long procedures on the cheek teeth, but the jaw should be closed every 15 minutes or so to give the jaw muscles a rest. The jaws are held open by seating the upper and lower incisors in incisor cups or rests that are mounted on the ends of upper and lower cheek pieces. For the comfort of the horse with severe brachygnathia, the upper incisor cup of the McPherson speculum can be replaced with a flat gum plate.

Full-mouth specula are available in different types of metal, designs, and sizes. The least expensive are made of nickel-plated cast iron or bronze alloys. The most expensive are stainless-steel. The straps that hold the speculum on also vary from inexpensive leather to premium-quality leather or high-quality synthetics, which are nearly indestructible.

Styles of specula that can be found are named after the designers. Both the McPherson and MacAllen specula are practically synonymous with the term full-mouth speculum because they have been the most common types used for many years. The two are similar in that they are large and heavy, held on with a halter, use a ratchet mechanism that allows the mouth to be opened to different widths, and have incisor cups. Several important differences exist between the two. The McPherson speculum has two spring-loaded ratchets, one on each side of the head. The MacAllen speculum has a single spring-less ratchet attached to the lower incisor plate. The incisor cups of the McPherson speculum are narrow and can bruise the gingiva caudal to the incisors. The MacAllen speculum has incisor cups that are wider and distribute the pressure over a greater area, which is less likely to cause bruising.

The McPherson speculum is made by many dental equipment manufacturers. The MacAllen speculum has been modified and is available from makers Meister or Conrad.

KEY POINT:

Even a heavily sedated horse can suddenly wake up and swing its head to look at ▶ something. A horse head with a full-mouth speculum attached can cause injury to the dentist or assistant. Constantly watch the horse for depth of sedation. Avoid sudden movements, some horses require a blind fold to keep them from reacting to movement.

■ ■ FLOATS

Floats are tools with a rough working surface, called a float blade, mounted on a handle. All floats are a type of rasp. The original floats were metal and had working surfaces somewhat similar to equine hoof rasps.

Equine dental floats have been in existence for more than 100 years with few changes in basic design until recently. The blades are available in several materials, including carbide chips, cutting surfaces of scored solid carbide, and carbide inserts with rotating cutting surfaces *(Fig. 2.8)*. The blades may be fixed to a flat or curved surface on the end of the shaft, or may be removable ones that can be resharpened or disposed. The handgrips are available in many materials and comfortable shapes. The shafts are long, short, straight, or bent at different angles. They are specialized for specific groups of teeth and even individual teeth *(Fig. 2.9)*(see *Box 2.2*). These modifications have improved floating efficiency dramatically.

Float Blades

The working surface of float blades are composed of either tungsten carbide chips bonded to a base or solid tungsten carbide that has been machine-scored to create file teeth.

Carbide-chips blades are not as sharp as solid carbide blades; however, if you replace blades often, they are still very effective. Carbide-chip blades are available in fine, medium, or coarse grit. The medium or coarse grit blades can be used to knock off sharp points before using the more expensive solid carbide blades. The fine grit is excellent for finish work. In contrast to solid carbide blades, which only cut in one direction, carbide-chip blades can be used in a push-and-pull manner. They are inexpensive and most are considered disposable unless bonded to a float, in which case the whole float must be sent in to have the blade regritted.

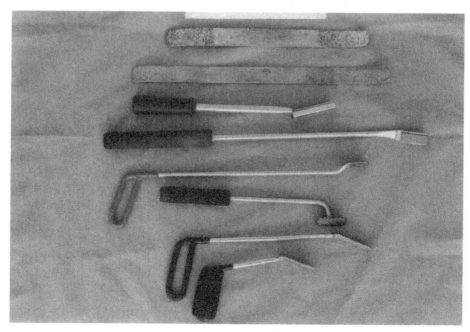

Figure 2.8   A collection of various types of floats from different manufacturers.

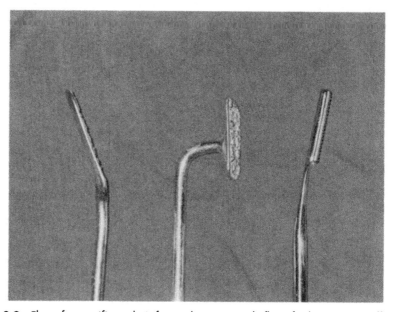

Figure 2.9   Floats for specific teeth. Left to right: open angle float, for lower #11s; offset float, for bit seats; closed angle float, for upper #11s.

BOX 2.2   FLOATS AND THEIR USES

Long straight float (solid carbide blade set on push): Lingual edges lower arcade and buccal edges #7, 8, 9 upper arcade.

Long straight float (solid carbide blade set on pull): Buccal edges upper #10.

Long obtuse float (solid carbide blade set on push): Blade surface of obtuse float is set at a greater than 90° angle (also called an open-angle float) relative to shaft. Angle varies according to preference. Buccal points upper arcade teeth #6–9.

Long closed-angle float: Blade surface is set at a less than 90° angle relative to shaft. Used to float the caudal surface of upper #11s.

Offset float: Bit seats on upper arcade.

Short open-angle float: Bit seats on lower arcade, finish work on upper #6–7.

Offset float (carbide-chip blade): Finish floating on upper #6–9.

S floats: Finish floating on caudal corner of 311 or 411, finish floating on buccal or lingual edges, finish work on teeth in which excess crown has been removed.

Small S floats or files: Finish work on canines or bit seats.

Solid carbide float blades are extremely sharp and very effective for removing tooth material. Solid carbide blades are also available in fine, medium, and coarse cutting blades. The coarser the blade, the more tooth material it removes. Very coarse blades get dull faster and are more likely to "chatter" or bounce over the teeth instead of cutting them. Medium and fine blades are easier to work with and remain sharp longer. They can be resharpened many times, whereas the coarse blades cannot because a considerable amount of metal is removed with each use.

KEY POINT:
▶ A solid carbide blade is somewhat brittle and can be chipped or broken.

Just like files, solid carbide blades are machined to cut in one direction. For work in the anterior portion of the mouth, setting the blade for cutting action on the push direction works most effectively. Cutting on the pull motion works best in the posterior part of the mouth because there is so little room to work, especially when working on the back molars.

Capps floats have blades that are made of three-sided carbide blade inserts that are pinned together to form a single unit *(Fig. 2.10)*. Because they have three working surfaces, the Capps floats give longer uninterrupted service than flat blades. However, they do not resharpen well and need to be replaced when dull. The Capps floats are extremely aggressive, compared to carbide burrs, in that they can remove a great amount of tooth material with just a few strokes.

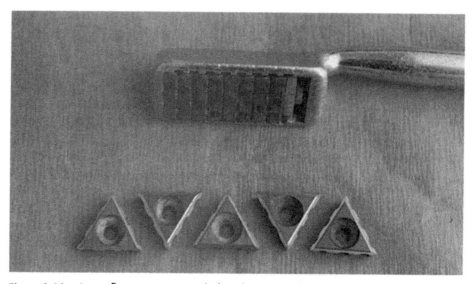

Figure 2.10 Capps floats are composed of stacking, 3-sided carbide inserts. These are very aggressive float blades.

S floats and incisor files do not have handles. S floats come in many sizes and are curved at both ends into an S shape. Both S floats and incisor files can have carbide chips or scored filing surfaces. The center of the float is the gripping area and has no filing surface. The smaller S floats are used to shape and smooth bit seats and to smooth canine teeth after they are cut. Large S floats, commonly called table floats, are used to float the lingual and buccal edges and to correct the occlusal surface of the most caudal maxillary teeth. Incisor files are short, straight files that are used to do finish off work on the incisors.

ELEVATORS, DENTAL PROBES, AND PICKS

Elevators are instruments used to elevate the gingiva surrounding a tooth. They are primarily used to facilitate extraction of wolf teeth, but may be used to elevate the tissue of any tooth within reach. Dental picks are also used as elevators when the gingiva surrounding a cheek tooth needs to be dissected from the tooth.

Wolf tooth elevators come in several styles and sizes *(Fig. 2.11)*. The most commonly used wolf tooth elevator is 6 or 7 inches long and is shaped like a short screw-driver with a half-moon blade. The curved half-moon shape allows the elevator to cup around the base of the tooth and dig under the gingiva into the alveolus. There are tubular elevators that look like large stainless steel biopsy punches that fit right over the entire wolf tooth. These elevators usually come in sets with interchangeable half-moon blades and tubular heads set at different angles. Pressure applied to the handle allows cutting completely around the tooth simultaneously with the tubular head. After the gingiva is cut, the half-moon elevator blade is used to elevate the root.

KEY POINT:
▶ When elevating the medial aspect of the wolf tooth, keep the elevator pressed firmly against the tooth to prevent it from slipping further medially where it could lacerate the palatine artery.

KEY POINT:
▶ Be sure to cut the gingiva completely away from the elevated tooth before removing it to prevent tearing a long strip of mucosa off the palate.

Dental picks are simple tools whose usefulness can be underestimated. The tips come in different shapes: needle point, lateral blade, and lingual blade *(Fig. 2.12)*. Most shapes are multipurpose and can be used to remove foreign material from between teeth, to elevate the gingiva prior to tooth extraction, or they can be wedged between teeth to loosen a tooth for extraction.

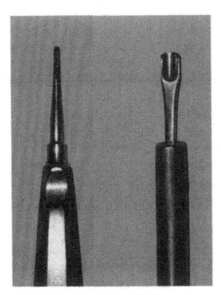

Figure 2.11 Small dental elevator (R) and half-moon wolf tooth elevator (L).

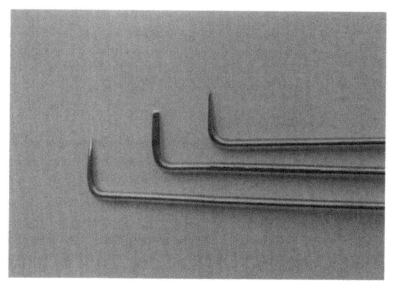

Figure 2.12   A set of dental probes (picks).

■ ■   MOLAR SPREADERS

This instrument is used to loosen molars to make them easier to extract orally. The cheek teeth are tightly packed together to create one long grinding surface out of each arcade. Disrupting this unity in order to remove one tooth is very difficult because there is no "wiggle room" between teeth. The molar spreaders are used to create a narrow space on either side of the tooth to be extracted by spreading and tearing the periodontal ligament. To operate the molar spreader, place the jaws between the mesial surface of the tooth to be extracted and the distal surface of the tooth rostral to it *(Fig. 2.13)*. Seat the jaws down about one-third of the height of the teeth, and squeeze until the blades of the jaw touch each other. Wiggle the spreaders loose, then place them another third deeper into this space and squeeze them shut again. Continue until the blades are just barely cutting through the gingival margin when you close them. After they are completely closed, tape the handles in the closed position. Support the closed handles for five minutes, then release and remove the spreaders. This is an effective way to breakdown periodontal attachments.

KEY POINT:
▶ Molar spreaders should be used cautiously when a #7 tooth is removed. Using them too aggressively in the mesial space can knock out tooth #6. Also, be careful not to bite too deeply into the gingiva when using molar spreaders on upper molars. The palatine artery lies in close proximity to the medial surface of these teeth.

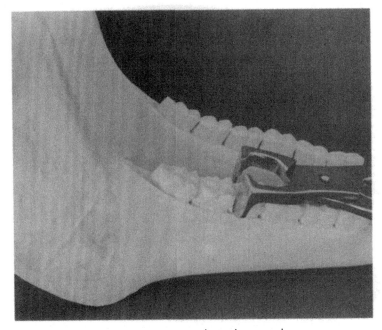

Figure 2.13 Seating the molar spreader.

■■ DENTAL FORCEPS

There are several types of dental forceps: incisor forceps, cap forceps, molar forceps, and root or fragment forceps. The main differences between these instruments are the size and shape of the head, and the length of the handles *(Fig. 2.14)*.

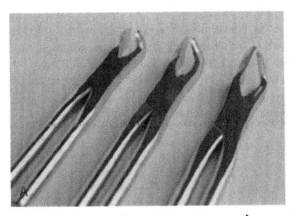
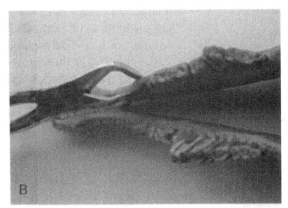

Figure 2.14 A. Forceps for removing incisors and tooth fragments of different sizes. B. Root fragment forceps in use. (Photographs courtesy of World Wide Equine.)

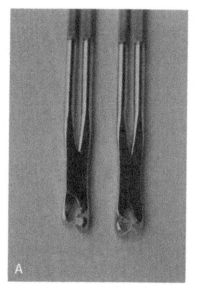
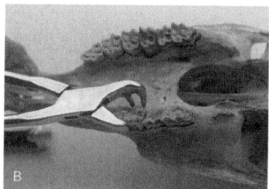

Figure 2.15   A. A set of Williams 3-root molar forceps. B. Correct positioning of the Williams 3-root molar forceps. Seat the double prongs in the mesial grooves of the tooth. (Photographs courtesy of World Wide Equine.)

Incisor forceps have narrow jaws for grasping the labial and lingual sides of incisors. Wolf tooth forceps are very similar to incisor forceps in size and shape and can be used to extract wolf teeth after they have been elevated, incisor caps, and premolar caps in miniature horses. Cap forceps, also known as cap extractors, are used to remove deciduous cheek teeth or permanent mandibular teeth that are loose or short-rooted. Some models have serrated jaws. Molar forceps are also called extractors. They are available in upper molar forceps and lower molar forceps. The jaw size is larger for upper molars and smaller for lower molars to facilitate a tight grip on just the tooth to be extracted. Williams 3-root molar forceps, made by World Wide Equine, are made for grasping molars with very little crown in aged horses *(Fig. 2.15 A and B)*. The three-prong design necessitates having a pair for use on the right side and a pair for the left side as well. The handles on molar forceps are approximately 22 inches long. Root fragment extractors have long narrow heads set at an angle to the handles. They are used to explore alveolar sockets for root fragments.

■ ■   **FULCRUMS**

Some sort of fulcrum may be needed to improve leverage when extracting molars *(Fig. 2.16)*. Extracting fulcrums are available in dental equipment catalogs. The problem is that sometimes the fulcrums are not the right size or shape, so you may need to improvise with pieces of wood or plastic to get just the right leverage.

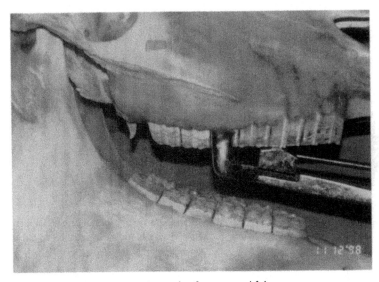

Figure 2.16 Molar forceps and fulcrum.

MOLAR CUTTERS

Molar cutters are a fast way to reduce long teeth. The tooth must need at least ¼ inch cut off or there will not be enough tooth to cut. The ideal situation is one is which the tooth shears along a plane that is parallel to the blades of the cutter. This is influenced by the internal resistance of the tooth material and will vary with the age of the tooth, the configuration of the enamel, and the density of the dentine and cementum components.

You need to understand two important things before using molar cutters. First, a level molar table is essential to using molar cutters correctly. Perform your floating and equilibration first. The cutters must be used parallel to a flat molar table. If you try to cut a tooth using an uneven molar surface to lay your cutters on, you may cut out a piece of jaw bone or fracture the tooth—both of which may make the jaw susceptible to bacterial infection. Second, molar cutters are designed to shear the tooth by exerting uniform pressure along the cutting surface. The only way to accomplish this is to use cutters with a head large enough or small enough to fit flush to as much of the tooth as possible. If you try to use a head that is too small, forcing the cutters to operate using a scissors action, you risk fracturing the tooth or breaking the cutters.

There are two basic types of molar cutters: simple joint and compound joint cutters. Within those types are cutters for teeth of varying widths. Simple joint cutters were designed to cut incisors, small molars, and hooks on molars (*Fig. 2.17 A and B*). Compound action cutters are powerful enough to cut the larger upper molars. The compound action provides significantly more leverage and sheering force to the cut-

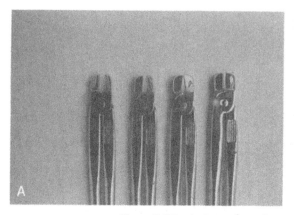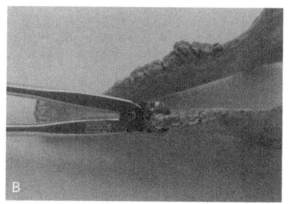

Figure 2.17   A. A set of simple joint molar cutters. (Photograph courtesy of World Wide Equine.) B. Using the D-head simple joint molar cutter to cut a mandibular tooth.

ting blades *(Fig. 2.18 A and B).* A complete set of molar cutters would be one compound cutter to cut long maxillary teeth and four simple molar cutters *(Table 2.1).*

The molar cutter is introduced into the mouth and positioned on the desired tooth with the handles level with the arcade. An assistant pulls the tongue to one side so that it is not caught between the cutting blades or the handles. The handles are closed

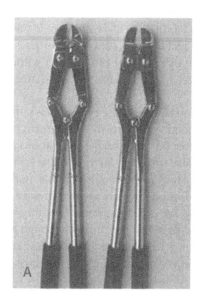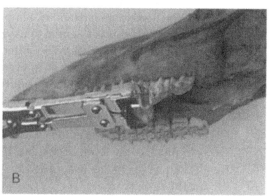

Figure 2.18   A. Thirty-degree open-head compound joint molar cutter for cutting excess crown from upper cheek teeth #6 and #7 (*left*). Zero-degree compound joint molar cutter (*right*). B. Correct positioning for cutting excess crown from an upper cheek tooth with the compound joint molar cutters. (Photographs courtesy of World Wide Equine.)

TABLE 2.1   Cutter Types

Type	Usage
Compound cutter	Maxillary teeth
A-head simple cutter	Small hooks on small mandibular #6s
B-head simple cutter	Small hooks on mandibular #11s
C-head simple cutter	Larger hooks on mandibular #11s
D-head cutter simple cutter	Mandibular teeth

onto the tooth to grasp it, and positioning is checked. If the cutter blades have not slipped out of position, the handles are firmly squeezed until the tooth is cut through.

■ ■   EQUI-CHIP

The Equi-Chip is a precision percussion dental chisel. A tap of the sliding percussion bolt hammers a hardened carbon steel blade to cut off second premolar and rear molar hooks. This instrument works best for rear hooks; however, the Curve of Spee may interfere with accurate positioning on the lower ones. It is difficult to position on the second premolar hooks (#6s), especially the lower ones. Dentists who use this instrument say that using a file to score the cut on #6 teeth will help seat the instrument more securely. The handle and blade must be elevated at a 45° angle to cut the hook properly, or you risk shearing off half the tooth.

To use this type of cutter on a #11 hook, position the blade on the caudal aspect of the hook and pull the sliding handle out in a quick, snapping motion, which causes the chisel to cut through the hook.

The Equi-Chip should not be used on teeth with cavities or in geriatric patients. Teeth with cavities may not shear in a predictable manner, and short-rooted geriatric teeth may be knocked out instead of cut.

KEY POINT:
▶ Accurate positioning is vital when using the Equi-Chip. If the instrument slips and the chisel strikes in an undesirable place, too much of the tooth could be sheared off or the tooth could fracture.

■ ■   MOTOR-DRIVEN EQUIPMENT

The introduction of motor-driven equipment revolutionized equine dentistry by removing much of the physical strength and endurance previously required to be a dentist. Many veterinarians who realized the need for dentistry in their equine patients were disappointed and frustrated by the inefficiency of the carbide-chip hand floats, making them reluctant to offer dentistry as a service. The motor drives a flexible shaft that attaches to a handpiece. In effect, these floats are heavy-duty versions of the motorized equipment used by dentists who treat humans. Motors should be operated with a variable speed control; the most common is the foot-operated control.

Currently there are three types of motorized dental instruments: power-driven floats that operate in a reciprocating (back-and-forth) fashion; rotary instruments mounted in handpieces attached to flexible shafts; and rotary instruments in which a carbide-chip disk rotates on the end of a solid shaft attached to the motor. Motorized equipment must be used on an adequately sedated animal in an uncluttered work area. The animal's head must be supported with a headstand or suspended from a dental halter. Although it is safer to use an assistant to help steady the head and re-

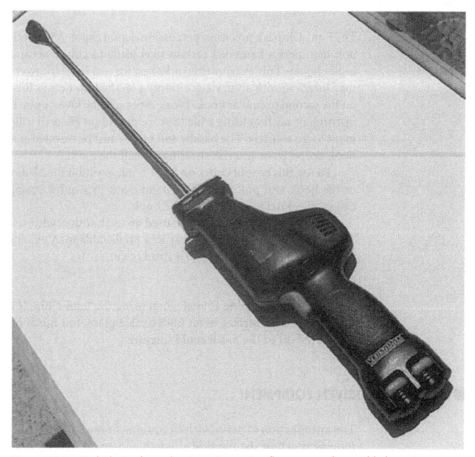

Figure 2.19 Carbide Products electric reciprocating float uses rechargeable batteries. (Photograph courtesy of Carbide Products.)

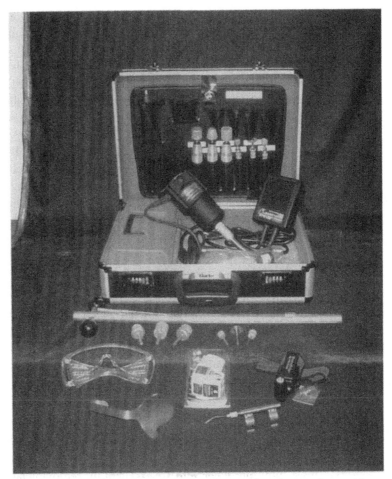

Figure 2.20 Heavy-duty electric Dremel operated rotary float kit manufactured by Equi-Dent.

tract the lips and tongue, it is possible to work solo if the horse is in stocks. Bungee cords or other forms of mechanical retractors can be used to retract soft tissue.

The reciprocating floats consist of a motor to which floats of different lengths and head shapes can be attached. Either carbide-chip or solid carbide blades can be used in these units. The stroke length varies according to the manufacturer. There are both electric and battery-operated units available *(Fig. 2.19)*.

Motors

The Dremel model 7 heavy-duty, .5-horsepower motor is the workhorse used by most equine dentists. Most likely, you will need to order it directly from Dremel or from an equine dental equipment supplier because it is hard to find in hardware or hobby stores that carry the smaller Dremel motors (see Appendix B at the back of the book). This motor has one speed, so it cannot be slowed down or sped up unless a variable-speed foot pedal or some sort of reostat is used. Dremel has a variable-speed foot pedal for this purpose *(Fig. 2.20)*.

World Wide Equine carries Metabo motors models 110 and 240. These motors have several features that make them different from the Dremel motors. A foot pedal or reostat speed control is not necessary because a variable speed feature is built into the motor unit. Handpieces are not needed either because burrs are attached directly to the shaft.

Carbide Products offers the Suhner motor model USC 9R that is made in Germany. This motor features 4000 to 9000 rpm, .67 horsepower, variable speed control, and reduction gears. This motor can be used with a clutch attachment manufactured by Carbide Products *(Fig. 2.21)*. The clutch attachment has an adjustable torque control to limit soft-tissue damage should the burr come into contact with mucosa.

Jupiter Veterinary Products also sells flexible-shaft rotary grinders.

Handpieces

Handpieces are required to attach the burrs or cutting wheels to the shaft of the Dremel and Suhner motors. The Dremel handpieces have enclosed bearing assemblies that can be replaced as the bearings wear out. The Dremel 1-inch Heavy-Duty handpiece is used for burrs with ¼-inch shafts. The Dremel ½-inch handpiece is used for attachments with ⅛-inch or ³⁄₃₂-inch shafts.

Burrs

Solid carbide and carbide-chip burrs are available in several sizes, lengths, shapes, and cutting patterns *(Box 2.3)*. Many companies offer resharpening and regritting services to extend the life of the burrs. Cylindrical, round, and conical burrs are the most common shapes and are excellent for removing large amounts of tooth material in a short time. The introduction of burrs with 8-inch to 12-inch shafts has virtually eliminated the need for using molar cutters to reduce long teeth in the posterior areas of the mouth *(Fig. 2.22)*.

Burr Guards and Extensions. A major concern when using motor-driven burrs is damage to soft tissue. This problem can be virtually eliminated by using clutch attachments to the motor and by using burr guards. There are many excellent burr guards on the market that attach to the handpiece to partially shield the tongue and cheek tissue *(Fig. 2.23)*. Burr guards are available in lengths corresponding to burr lengths. Carbide Products makes a 12-inch burr guard with a vacuum channel that aspirates tooth dust as it cuts *(Fig. 2.24)*. Equi-Dent makes a guarded burring instrument, called the caudal hook grinder, with a long, small-diameter extension handle that allows excellent visualization while reducing #11 teeth. World Wide Equine also makes burr guards that are attached to extension handles.

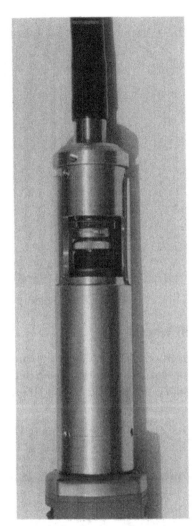

Figure 2.21   Suhner motor unit with slip clutch attachment between motor and flex shaft to prevent soft-tissue damage. (Photograph courtesy of Carbide Products.)

BOX 2.3   BURRS AND CUT-OFF WHEELS

$\frac{1}{2}$-inch round burr: Solid carbide or carbide chip.
$\frac{5}{8}$-inch round burr: Solid carbide or carbide chip.
Carbide-chip conical burr.
Carbide-chip bit seat burr.
Oblong burr: set on an 8–12-inch shaft; Solid carbide.
Diamond cut-off wheels: available in $\frac{3}{4}$-inch to $1\frac{5}{8}$-inch diameter.

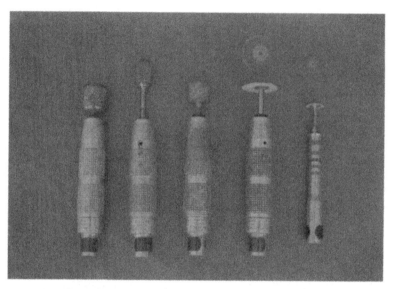

Figure 2.22   Rotary burrs and diamond cutoff wheels.

Cut-Off Wheels

Cut-off wheels are coated with diamond dust on both sides of the wheel. They are ideal for scoring and cutting teeth in the anterior aspect of the mouth, especially incisors and canines. In addition to their cutting action, they can also be used to grind

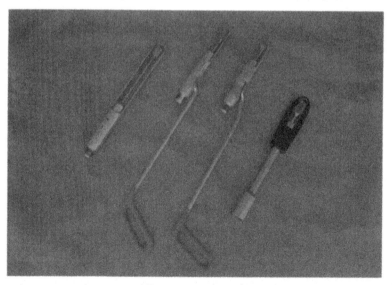

Figure 2.23   Burr guards come in different lengths and shapes depending on the area of the mouth in which they are to be used.

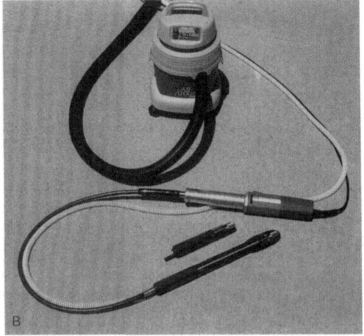

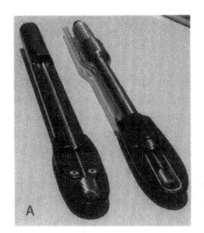

Figure 2.24 A. 12-inch GT handpiece with titanium-coated, double-cut burr (*left*) and 12-inch Dremel guard with external vacuum chamber (*right*). B. 12-inch handpiece, 4-inch incisor handpiece, heavy duty flex shaft, and drive unit with clutch. 12-inch Dremel guard with vacuum attaches to a wet/dry, low-noise vacuum and vacuum line. (Equipment by Carbide Products.)

off tooth material. Diamond wheels are available in 1-inch diameter on a ⅛-inch shaft and 1⅝-inch diameter on a ¼-inch shaft.

Rotary Floats

At this writing, there are two companies manufacturing electric power floats, Swissvet (Swissfloat) and D and B Enterprises (Powerfloat). Both of these instruments have a rotating grinding disk set at a 45° angle on the end of a long rigid shaft and can be used for both incisor and cheek teeth reduction. The head profile of the Powerfloat is low enough to allow work on the difficult upper #11s *(Fig. 2.25 A* and *B)*.

Pneumatic Floats

Pneumatic floats, or air rasps, operate in a reciprocating manner, driven by compressed air *(Fig. 2.26)*. Stubbs Equine Innovations makes a remotely located compressor with a minimum output of 4 cfm at 90 psi used to drive the float head.

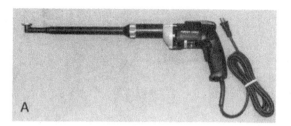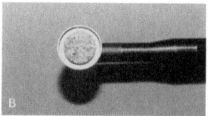

Figure 2.25 A. The Power Float. (Photograph courtesy of D & B Enterprises.) B. Close-up of the rotary grinding disk of the Power Float.

Pneumatic floats move forward and backward at speeds of 9,000 to 10,000 oscillations per minute. The stroke is short, 3/8-inch (10 mm), which makes the float safe for use on the third molars (#11s). All the teeth, including incisors and canines, can be floated or reduced in height using handpieces of different lengths and angles. The handpieces are light, trigger-operated, and easily interchangable. Olson and Silk also offer a pneumatic float kit.

There are several advantages to using pneumatic floats instead of rotary instruments. A polymer lubricant can be used to reduce heat produced by friction. The lubricant also reduces production of airborne dust. Electric shock from using power instruments in a wet environment is not a problem. Finally, there are no moving parts to become clogged with tooth dust.

Portable Stocks for Dentistry

A mobile equine stock is available from Stubbs Equine Innovations. The stock folds down for transport and moves into an upright working position using a hydraulic mechanism.

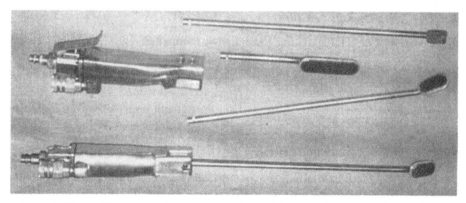

Figure 2.26 Stubbs air rasp hand units and floats. (Photograph courtesy of Dr. Stubbs.)

■■ EQUIPMENT CLEANING AND MAINTENANCE

Dentistry equipment is expensive, and many instruments eventually wear out, requiring replacement. To prolong the useful life of your instruments, you should clean and inspect them for damage after each use. This will prevent having to deal with broken or unusable equipment while at your next appointment.

Speculums

Wash off tooth dust and blood using antiseptic soap; then dry. Inspect bolts in full-mouth speculums for any indication of looseness. If possible, store speculums in their own padded bag or container.

Floats

Scrub the tooth dust out of the blades with a fine, copper-wire brush. Inspect solid carbide blades for dullness and chipping. Wash the handle and handgrip, then dry them or lay them out to dry. Store floats so that the blades are protected. Have several sets of new or resharpened blades on hand at all times. Carbide chip 5-files and floats need to be sent to the manufacturer to be re-surfaced when dull.

Burrs and Handpieces

Scrub tooth dust out of burrs using a stiff toothbrush. Check burrs and wheels for dullness and damage. Do not immerse handpieces, but wipe them clean. Spin burrs and cutoff wheels while they are attached to the handpieces by flipping them with a finger to inspect for bent shafts, bent wheels, and signs of the bearings wearing out. Burrs and wheels should spin fluidly and effortlessly, with no signs of resistance or wobbling. If there is resistance, the handpiece needs to have bearings replaced. If there is wobble in the action of the burr or wheel, remove it and inspect it for a bent shaft or wheel. Have new burrs and diamond wheels on hand to replace dull ones immediately. This will help reduce strain on your motor and to reduce heat production on the teeth you are remodeling.

Motors and Flex Shafts

Wipe case clean. Periodically remove flex shafts, and apply a light layer of shaft grease. At this time, you can also check the motor brushes for signs of excess wear. Keep a copy of the parts list for the motor and shaft in a sealed sandwich bag with your motor in case you need to call the manufacturer. Always have a spare motor, shaft, and handpieces on hand, and repair broken equipment immediately *(Fig. 2.27)*.

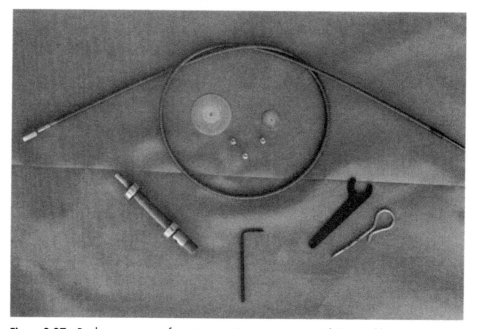

Figure 2.27 Replacement parts for rotary equipment are essential. Pictured here is a spare cable for the Dremel flex shaft, the enclosed bearings unit for a large Dremel handpiece, spare set screws for burr guards, diamond cut-off wheels, and a Dremel wrench set.

Other Instruments

Clean and inspect for wear and damage.

■ ■ SUGGESTED READINGS

Easley J. Dental Care and Instrumentation. Veterinary Clinics of North America Equine Practice. Philadelphia: WB Saunders, 1998.

Scrutchfield WL. Equine dental instrumentation. In: Baker GJ, Easley J, eds. Equine Dentistry. Philadelphia: WB Saunders, 1999.

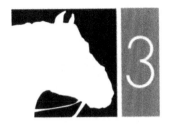

THE DENTAL EXAMINATION

PATRICIA PENCE

Dental disease has been underrecognized as a cause of health and behavior problems in horses. Comprehensive oral examinations were not frequently performed because veterinarians and owners assumed the incidence of dental abnormalities to be low. However, recent surveys have shown abnormal dentition to be more common than previously thought. A survey by Uhlinger showed that 24% of young horses, with and without symptoms, had dental abnormalities.[1] In a comprehensive study of skulls of slaughtered horses, Kirkland and colleagues found that more than 80% of 500 skulls showed evidence of oral disease or dental pathology.[2] Cheek teeth abnormalities are the least likely to be discovered without a comprehensive oral examination, but were found by Dixon and colleagues to be the most common.[3,4,5,6] In a review of 400 horses referred because of dental disorders, 44 cases suffered from primary disorders of the incisors, 11 from disorders of canine or wolf teeth, and 345 from primary disorders of cheek teeth. See *Table 3.1* for examples of age-related dental abnormalities.

Presently, dental examinations are becoming an accepted component of equine preventative health care, bringing attention to the variety of dental disease in apparently asymptomatic horses. We have recognized a great need exists for more studies concerning equine dental anatomy, physiology, pathology, and possible methods of treatment.

This chapter will introduce topics related to the dental examination: safety issues, sedation, equipment needed, the importance of a detailed history, examination of external features, evaluation of condition, the oral examination, common and age-related dental abnormalities, and charting.

TABLE 3.1   Age-related Dental Abnormalities[1-7]

Age	Type of Abnormality
Birth to 2 years	Congenital/Developmental Defects
	Parrot-mouth (prognathism)
	Sow-mouth (brachynathism)
	Wry-nose (pre-maxilla and mandible deviated laterally)
	Missing teeth (with or without overgrowth of opposing teeth)
	Supernumerary teeth (with or without crowding of surrounding teeth)
	Caudal displacement of mandibular arcades (hooks or ramps on 106, 206)
	Rostral displacement of mandibular arcades (hooks or ramps on 306, 406)
	Developmental cysts
	Neoplasia
	Trauma
	Fractures
	Avulsed incisors
	Crowded deciduous incisors
	Sharp enamel points
	Impacted (blind) wolf teeth
2½ to 5 years	Developmental Problems
	Caudial displacement of mandibular arcades (hooks or ramps on 106, 206, possibly on 311, 411)
	Rostral displacement of mandibular arcades (hooks or ramps on 306, 406, possibly on 111, 211)
	Eruption Problems
	Delayed shedding of deciduous teeth (retained caps)
	Premature eruption of permanent teeth
	Impacted cheek teeth
	Crowded permanent incisors
	Eruption cysts or pseudocysts
	Overgrown Incisors
	Trauma
	Fractures, of jaw or tooth
	Avulsed incisors
	Trauma-related injury to immature root
	Infection
	Periostitis
	Sharp enamel points (with or without associated soft-tissue abrasions and lacerations)
	Canine tooth impactions
5 to 20 years	Neoplasia
	Deviations in Occlusal Contact
	Wave mouth
	Step mouth
	Sheer mouth
	Caudal and rostral mandibular displacement and associated overgrown corner cheek teeth as described above
	Overgrown or abnormally worn incisors
	Long, sharp canines
	Tartar accumulation
	Trauma (as described above)
	Gingivitis and periodontal disease
	Caries
	Tooth loss (with or without overgrowth of opposing tooth)

TABLE 3.1   *Continued*

Age	Type of Abnormality

Older than 20 years	Tooth displacement (secondary to stress from abnormal wear or tooth loss)
	Sharp enamel points (with or without associated soft tissue abrasions and lacerations)
	Deviations in occlusal contact as above
	Caries, sagittally fractured maxillary teeth
	  Tooth loss (with overgrowth of opposing tooth)
	Tooth displacement as described above
	Cupped occlusal surface of cheek teeth
	Overgrown or abnormally worn incisors
	Gingivitis and periodontal disease
	  Metaplastic calicification
	Cracked and broken teeth
	  Sharp enamel edges
	  Neoplasia

The purpose of the equine dental examination is to determine whether a pathologic condition exists and to evaluate the effect of that condition on the horse's overall health and comfort. Once such a condition is identified, a treatment plan can then be proposed to correct and manage the condition. In addition, an estimate of costs must be determined for the owner/client.

■ ■ SAFETY ISSUES AND CHEMICAL RESTRAINT

The dental examination and dental procedures must be performed in an area safe for the practitioner, the assistant, and the horse (see *Box 3.1* for a list of necessary equipment). The area must be free of objects such as wheelbarrows, rakes, wood piles, blankets, feed and water buckets, and water hoses. Also, ensure that children and pets are not in the area. Working on the horse in a set of stocks is ideal but not always possible. Positioning the horse with its hindquarters in the corner of a stall or a pen will help prevent the horse from walking backward and provide posterior stabilization after the horse is sedated. Practitioners that prefer to support the head with a dental halter put the horse in a stall or other doorway if a method of anchoring the rope above the horse's head is available. Neither the practitioner nor the assistant should be in a position that could trap them with an agitated or violent horse, should that occur.

Animals typically resent having humans stick fingers into their mouths, and horses are no exception. Examiners must be aware that a horse can rear or strike them or their assistant with a foreleg; thus, constant attention to the mood of the horse being examined is imperative. Learn to watch for signs of fear, anger, or frus-

---

BOX 3.1   EQUIPMENT FOR DENTAL EXAMINATION

Adjustable halter and lead rope
Dental halter (padded metal noseband) and rope
Full-mouth speculum
Light
Dental picks
Cheek retractors
Bucket of dilute antiseptic
Dose syringe
Hand towel or paper towels
Flexible fiberoptic endoscope (if available)
Timer

---

tration and to recognize softening and relaxation. If the horse does not relax or at least tolerate your initial examination, sedate the horse for the safety of yourself, your assistant, and the horse. Sedation is more humane for the horse and more reassuring for the owner than physical restraint.

Detomidine, xylazine, and butorphanol are excellent sedatives for dental examinations and procedures.[7] Detomidine and butorphanol produce less ataxia and are longer-acting medications. Xylazine is a shorter-acting medication, and is less expensive. However, it is more likely to cause ataxia or recumbency at higher doses.[8] A commonly used mixture is 0.5 mg/kg xylazine plus 2 ug/kg detomidine HCl or 0.5mg/kg butorphanol at the start of the procedure, with injection of small amounts (0.5–0.75 mg/kg) of xylazine as needed to prolong sedation.[7] All horses are different in their tolerance of sedatives. Usually, a gentle, calm horse will require smaller amounts of sedatives than one that is fearful, suspicious, or stubbornly resistant. Ponies and miniature horses sometimes require a higher dose than an average-sized (500kg) horse. Draft horses may need a lower dose than expected for their size.

KEY POINT:

▶ Wait 5 minutes for the sedative to take effect before putting in the speculum. Use a kitchen or laboratory timer to ensure that you wait the full 5 minutes.

PRACTICE TIP:

A common side effect of butorphanol is that the horse leans forward heavily, even to the point of stumbling or walking toward the practitioner. In such cases, the use of a headstand is impossible, so use this drug sparingly, suspend the head in a dental halter, or restrain the horse in stocks.

BOX 3.2   CLINICAL SIGNS ASSOCIATED WITH DENTAL DISEASE

Losing weight in spite of good appetite
Failure to gain weight
Dribbling grain
Obvious chewing abnormalities
Signs of facial tenderness
Accumulating wads of grass or hay between the buccal gingiva and the cheek teeth (quidding)
Soaking hay in water before eating it
Drooling
Foul breath
Excessive whole grain particles in feces
Roughage particles longer than $\frac{1}{4}$ inch in feces
Discharge from nostrils
Fistulous discharge from the jaw or face
Swelling on the lower jaw or face

■ ■   SIGNALMENT AND HISTORY

The horse's age, sex, breed, and description need to be recorded. Useful information to include in a thorough history is vaccination records, deworming program, prior and current medical problems, reproductive status, use of the horse, and vices or behavioral problems. See *Box 3.2* for clinical signs and *Box 3.3* for behavior or performance problems that may be associated with dental disease.

It is important to note any medical conditions that may be complicated if the horse is sedated, stressed, or traumatized by an extensive dental procedure. Xylazine and detomidine can cause severe bradycardia with an associated decrease in cardiac output, which may be dangerous in a horse with cardiac disease.[9] Horses with car-

---

BOX 3.3   PERFORMANCE OR BEHAVIOR SIGNS ASSOCIATED WITH DENTAL DISEASE

Head tossing
Rearing
Fighting the bit
Refusal to take the bit
Refusal to take a lead
Race horses lugging in or out on the turns
Harness horses not staying in frame
Barrel horses refusing to make tight turns or failure to complete a turn

---

diac disease, including arrhythmias, may require a predental workup and the administration of medications to stabilize the heart prior to sedation. Horses with liver or kidney disease may require a lower dose of sedative, or sedatives not excreted by the impaired organ. Horses with liver disease may also have blood-clotting problems that could create excessive blood loss if teeth are extracted. Horses with pituitary adenomas are more susceptible to infection and may need predental antibiotics to fight bacterial invasion of mucosal abrasions.

Whenever the oral mucosa is interrupted, a transient bacteremia can occur, and one should be expected when an abscessed tooth is extracted. Use of predental antibiotics should be considered, especially for geriatric animals with periodontal disease. Horses recovering from surgery or experiencing active inflammation of joints should not have dental procedures performed until healing has occurred and inflammation has subsided. The risk of bacterial colonization of areas of inflammation should be considered against the risk of adverse events if the dental procedure is postponed.

As with many medical procedures, appropriate client communication is the best way to prevent misunderstandings. This is particularly important if something does not go as planned. Obtaining written consent from the client before performing dental procedures will remind you to inform the client adequately of risks that may be involved.

For a horse being examined because the client believes there is a problem, a thorough history regarding the problem is important. For example, if the horse has been losing weight, determine what it is being fed, how much it is being fed, whether the owner/client is consistently weighing food portions, and how hard the horse is being worked. It is important to know if the horse did not shed well the previous spring, has increased thirst or urination, tires easily, or has a chronic cough, nasal discharge, or chronic diarrhea.

KEY POINT:
▶ Rule out other causes of weight loss such as parasites, organ dysfunction, internal abscesses, neurologic deficits, maldigestion/malabsorption problems, pulmonary disease, or cardiac disease if the oral conditions found during the dental examination do not correlate with the overall condition of the horse.

■ ▦ EXAMINING EXTERNAL FEATURES

A physical examination of the external features of the horse's body should be performed. The fleshiness of the body and condition of the horse's coat should be recorded. See *Figure 3.1* and *Box 3.4* for information about assigning condition scores.

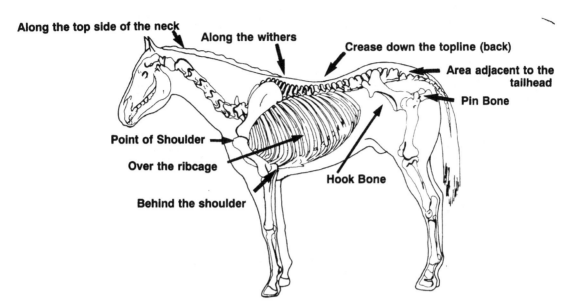

Along the top side of the neck

Along the withers

Crease down the topline (back)

Area adjacent to the tailhead

Pin Bone

Point of Shoulder

Over the ribcage

Hook Bone

Behind the shoulder

Figure 3.1   Areas of interest in body condition evaluation. Reprinted with permission from Robert A. Mowrey, Extension Horse Husbandry Specialist, North Carolina Cooperative Extension Service.

Stand back and examine the face and head of the horse. Is the horse's attitude alert and calm, anxious and fearful, or dull and nonresponsive? Check for symmetry of the muscles of mastication, that is, the temporal and massetar muscles, the nostrils, the lips, and the eyelids (**Fig. 3.2**). Are the eyes level and symmetrical? Look for facial swellings, muscle atropy or hypertrophy, abnormal facial expressions, draining tracts, and nasal discharge (**Figs. 3.3, 3.4, 3.5**). If there is a nasal discharge, check for objectionable odor. Also check the saliva and breath for odor.

Gently palpate the facial features associated with mastication to detect pain or swelling: the temporomandibular joint, the superficial facial nerves, the temporal and massetar muscles, and the edges of the upper cheek teeth. Pay attention to the horse's reaction when you press the tissue over the enamel edges of the last upper cheek teeth (#111 and 211). It is common for horses to tolerate palpation of the other cheek teeth, then react painfully to pressure over the last upper cheek teeth because the skin is drawn tighter over these teeth, which can create buccal abrasions and ulcers.

KEY POINT:
▶ When dental procedures are done at the stable, check the horse's pen or stall for signs of abnormal mastication, such as hay quids, pools of saliva, excess grain on the ground, and hay in the water trough. Examine the feces for consistency, moisture content, and presence of undigested grain, noting the size of undigested roughage particles.

BOX 3.4   A PRACTICAL SYSTEM FOR ASSIGNING BODY CONDITION SCORES TO HORSES

Condition	Neck	Withers	Loin	Tailhead	Ribs	Shoulder
1 POOR	Bone structure noticeable	Bone structure easily noticeable	Spinous processes project prominently	Tailhead, pin bones, and hook bones project prominently	Project prominently	Bone structure easily noticeable
2 VERY THIN	Faintly discernible Animal emaciated	Faintly discernible	Slight fat covering over base of spinous processes; transverse processes of lumbar vertebrae feel rounded; spinous processes are prominent	Prominent	Prominent	Faintly discernible
3 THIN	Accentuated	Accentuated	Fat buildup halfway on spinous processes, but easily discernible; transverse processes cannot be felt	Tailhead prominent, but individual vertebrae cannot be visually identified; hook bones appear rounded, but are still easily discernible; pin bones not distinguishable	Slight fat cover over ribs; ribs easily discernible	Accentuated

	Neck	Withers	Back	Tailhead	Ribs	Shoulder
4 MODERATELY THIN	Not obviously thin	Not obviously thin	Negative crease along back	Prominence depends on conformation; fat can be felt; hook bones not discernible	Faint outline discernible	Not obviously thin
5 MODERATE	Blends smoothly into body	Rounded over spinous processes	Back level	Fat around tailhead beginning to feel spongy	Cannot be visually distinguished, but can be easily felt	Blends smoothly into body
6 MODERATELY FLESHY	Fat beginning to be deposited	Fat beginning to be deposited	May have slight positive crease down back	Fat around tailhead feels soft	Fat over ribs feels spongy	Fat beginning to be deposited; point-of-shoulder not discernible
7 FLESHY	Fat deposited along neck	Fat deposited along withers	May have positive crease down back behind shoulder	Fat around tailhead is soft	Individual ribs can be felt, but noticeable filling between ribs with fat	Fat deposited behind shoulder
8 FAT	Noticeable thickening of neck Fat deposited along inner buttocks	Area along withers filled with fat	Positive crease down back	Tailhead fat very soft	Difficult to feel ribs	Area behind shoulder filled in, flush with body
9 EXTREMELY FAT	Bulging fat Fat along inner buttocks may rub together; flank filled in flush	Bulging fat	Obvious positive crease down back	Building fat around tailhead	Patchy fat appearing over ribs	Bulging fat

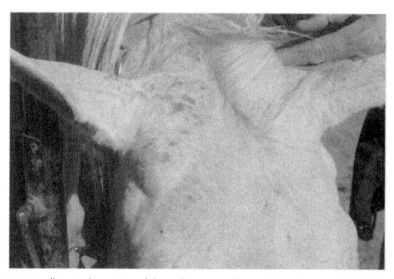

Figure 3.2 Swelling in the region of the right temporalis muscle in this grey horse was caused by melanoma infiltration. Do not assume all mastication muscle swelling results from dental disease.

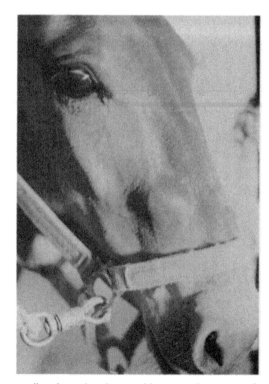

Figure 3.3 This firm swelling lateral to the nasal bones in the region of tooth #107 roots of this young horse could be owing to a developmental abnormality of dental, bone, or soft-tissue structures.

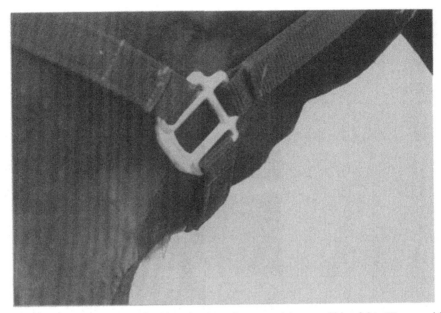

Figure 3.4 These paired swellings on the ventral aspect of the mandible of this 3½-year-old horse are at the site of developing tooth roots of #306, #307. These are commonly called eruption cysts.

■ ■ THE ORAL EXAMINATION

There are two types of oral examinations: (1) brief and cursory, and (2) thorough and methodical.

The Brief Dental Examination

The cursory examination is not an examination per se, but rather a brief inspection of the incisors, a peek at the first upper and lower cheek teeth, and mandibular manipulation to check occlusion (*Fig. 3.6*). Obviously not much information can be obtained from this type of examination. However, it does establish in the client's mind that dental care is important without altering the practitioner's and the client's schedules for the day.

To perform an examination of a horse's mouth without a sedative and a speculum, you must take a minute to gain the horse's trust and show that you do not intend any harm. Stroke the horse's cheeks, rub around the eyes, and finally work your way down to this muzzle. Rinse out any hay or grass with a dose syringe; otherwise, you will not be able to see beyond the incisors. Look for incisor abnormalities, wolf teeth, sharp enamel points, and hooks or ramps on the first upper and lower cheek

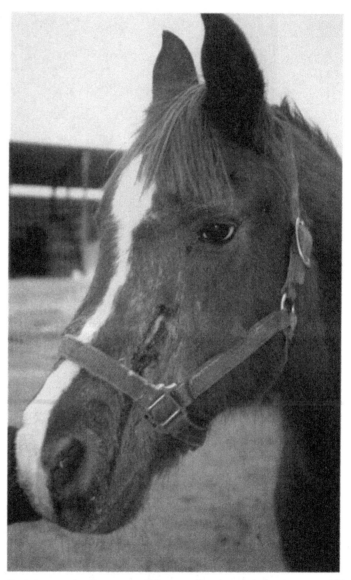

Figure 3.5   Draining tract in the region of the maxillary sinuses of a 25-year-old horse. Differential diagnoses would include trauma, primary sinus infection, tooth root infection, and neoplasia. Tooth root infection would be less likely to cause maxillary sinus drainage in a horse this age because the roots no longer lie within the floor of the sinuses. If this horse were younger, than 15 years, dental disease would be more plausible.

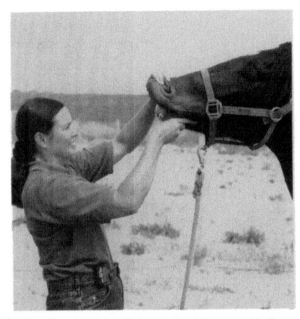

Figure 3.6 The brief oral examination of a cooperative horse would allow inspection of the incisors, wolf teeth and canines, and perhaps the first cheek teeth.

teeth (*Fig. 3.7*). Palpate the enamel edges of the upper #11s. Check molar occlusion by sliding the mandible laterally to one side and then the other (see description in the following). The practitioner can point out problems, such as sharp enamel points, overgrown teeth, incisor abnormalities, and lack of normal occlusion or excursion of the cheek teeth. However, if no problems become apparent during this inspection, the practitioner should still point out that this does not rule out forms of dental disease that can only be detected using a full-mouth speculum and a good source of light. The client should then be urged to make an appointment for a thorough oral examination at a more convenient time.

To check occlusion:

- Drop the horse's head into the position that the horse would hold it to chew its food. The poll should be at approximately the same level as the whithers.
- Stand to the side of the head with your ear close to the cheek (*Fig. 3.8*).
- Grasp the bridge of the nose with one hand and the ventral mandible with the other hand.
- Slide the mandible laterally to each side, listening and feeling for sounds and vibrations from the teeth. Discern whether the sounds emanate from the cheek teeth and incisors or whether all the sounds come from the incisors. In a normal horse, you should hear a soft grinding sound emanating from the cheek teeth evenly from both the posterior and the anterior teeth. The incisors

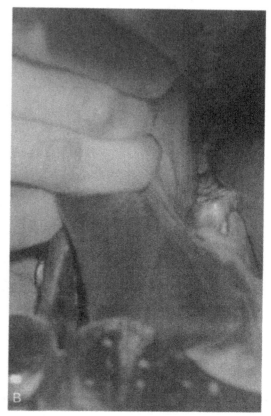

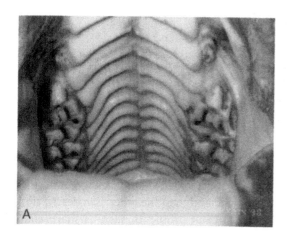

Figure 3.7 Wolf teeth abnormalities. A. Wolf teeth in abnormally rostral position. B. Wolf teeth in lower arcades are not commonly seen.

should make a smooth, sliding sound. Absence of sounds from areas you expect to hear them may indicate lack of occlusion.

To check lateral mandibular excursion:

- Stand in front of the horse with its head at normal chewing height.
- Cup the ventral muzzle in one hand and lift the upper lip with the other.
- Align the incisors directly over each other in the neutral position (*Fig. 3.9A*).
- Slowly slide the mandible laterally to one side, and note approximately how many millimeters you must move it before you can feel the cheek teeth on that side coming into contact with each other. Feel for unevenness of motion, which can indicate uneven teeth interlocking with each other (*Fig. 3.9B*).
- Determine whether the horse has to open its mouth for lateral excursion to occur (*Fig. 3.9C*).

- Repeat on the other side.
- Record millimeters of slide for each side.

The amount of lateral excursion is measured by the distance the central incisor on that side moves off the neutral position, i.e., how far does #401 move in relation to #101. Studies have yet to correlate distance of lateral excursion with degree of cheek teeth occlusion; however, a relation appears to exist.

Next, rub the upper and lower lips, occasionally sliding a fingertip between the lips. Once the horse tolerates the presence of your finger, you can palpate the gum tissue in the upper and lower interdental spaces for unerupted (blind) wolf teeth or canines. Work your way back to feel the buccal edges of the upper cheek teeth on both sides. You will only be able to feel the edges of the first one to three upper cheek teeth without a speculum. Check for foul odors.

Estimate the horse's age using eruption and wear patterns of the incisors. Check the incisors for retained deciduous teeth, broken teeth, missing teeth, supernumer-

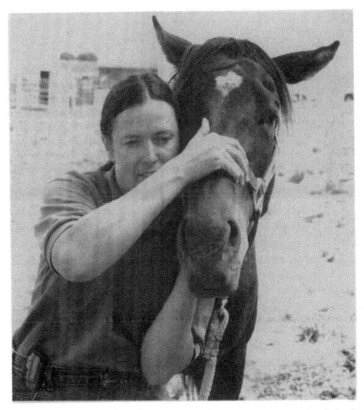

Figure 3.8   Identifying the location of occlusal noises is an important part of checking occlusion.

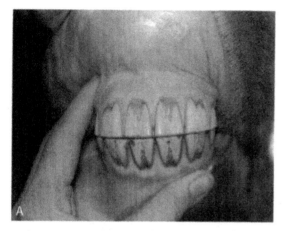

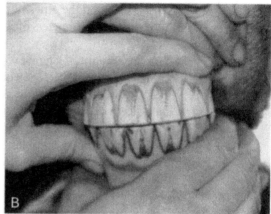

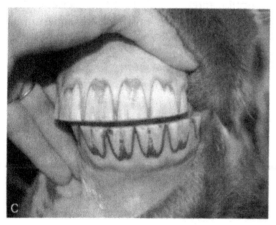

Figure 3.9 Checking lateral excursion. A. Align the incisors in neutral position. B. Slide the mandible to one side until you feel the cheek teeth come into contact. C. Dental abnormalities may force a horse to open its mouth to complete lateral excursion. D. In some horses, the incisors do not line up even when their jaws are in the neutral position. (Photographs by Kristin Wilewski. Used with permission.)

ary teeth, and evidence of cribbing or wood chewing (See Color Plates 1–9). Note the angle of eruption. The incisors continue to erupt and change from a primarily vertical eruption to a more proximally slanting one (***Fig. 3.10A,B***). Over time, this commonly creates an upward "smile" appearance, called a ventral curvature, to the incisors. Occasionally there is a dorsal curvature, that is, "frown" appearance, diagonal slant, or jagged line between the incisors (***Fig. 3.11A–D***). Currently, these are considered pathologic conditions that must be corrected. Even the upward smile must be made more horizontal if the incisors are preventing adequate molar occlusion.

If the horse has tolerated the procedures thus far, you can proceed to grasp the tongue for a look inside the mouth. Have an assistant hold a flashlight for you, or you can wear a headlamp. Pull the tongue out the side of the mouth through the interdental space with one hand then grasp the upper lip and pull it up with the other hand. Remember that the tongue is attached to the hyoid apparatus, so do not pull too powerfully. Look for hooks or ramps on both upper and lower second premolars, wolf teeth, wavy or step-like molar arcades, cupped molars, missing teeth, overgrown teeth, broken teeth, loose teeth, feed impacted in periodontal spaces, and gingivitis. Try to visualize the upper and lower caudal molars if you can, but this is not usually possible without using a speculum.

The Complete Dental Examination

Before the horse is sedated, check occlusion and lateral excursion as previously described.

After the horse is sedated, rinse the mouth thoroughly. Put in a full-mouth speculum making sure the incisors are well seated in the middle of the incisor cups. Tighten the poll strap enough to keep the horse from spitting out the speculum but not so tight that it interferes with work on the enamel points of the maxillary teeth. Adjust the nose strap, if present, to fit the horse.

PRACTICE TIP:

Doing a quick float to knock off the maxillary enamel points before you put in the speculum is a good idea. The speculum stretches the cheeks tight against these jagged points and may cause enough pain to prevent the horse from being sedated adequately.

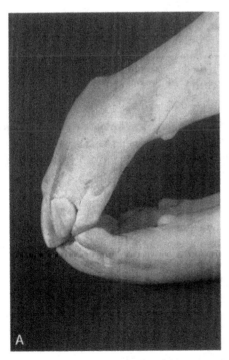
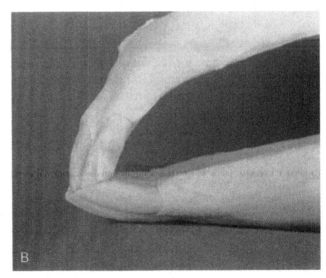

Figure 3.10 A. The angle of eruption in young horses is vertical. B. As more tooth erupts, the angle becomes more acute.

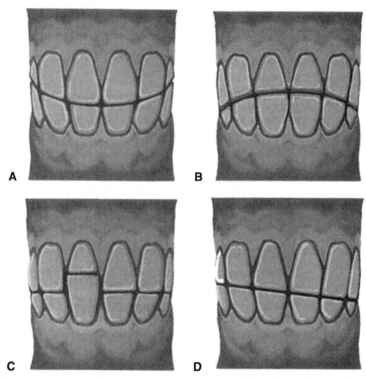

Figure 3.11   Classification of incisor malalignment. A. Smile misalignment. B. Frown misalignment. C. Step misalignment. D. Tilt or slant misalignment. (Reprinted with permission from Lowder MQ, Mueller PO. Dental disease in geriatric horses. In Dentistry, Gaughan EM, DeBowes RM, eds. Veterinary Clinics of North America. WB Saunders: Philadelphia, 1998.)

The sedative will cause the horse to drop its head too low to work on unless some sort of support is used. You can suspend the head using a rope attached to a metal-frame dental halter or attached to the speculum. Throw the rope over an overhead support such as a stall door frame (*Fig. 3.12*); or, if you prefer, use a headstand (*Fig. 3.13*).

Using direct light—either from a headlamp, flashlight, or halogen shop lamp—is imperative to visualize differences in tooth height, cracked teeth, caries, and food-filled gingival pockets. Examine the upper and lower caudal cheek teeth for hooks; the buccal gingiva for lacerations, ulcers, and calluses; and the tongue for lacerations (see Color Plates 10–27). Telescoping mechanics' mirrors and dental probes help visualization and exploration of areas in the mouth that are difficult to see (*Fig 3.14*). For magnified and comprehensive gingival examinations, the endoscope or intra-oral camera needed. Both can be used to search the oral cavity for the origin of fetid mouth odors. In cases in which foul-smelling exudate from the nostrils is present, the endoscope can be passed through the nostrils to study the nasal folds, ethmoid turbinates, pharynx, and gutteral pouches. A speculum must be used to protect the endoscope or intra-oral camera when either is in the oral cavity. Labial, occlusal, and buccal aspects of molars and gingiva can be closely examined for disease by using the magnifying and illuminating capabilities of these instruments. Retract the tongue and buccal cheek pockets away from the teeth to improve visibility.

For abnormal facial contours, such as swellings, bumps, draining tracts, and fractures, radiographs might need to be taken to determine the precise nature of the problem.[10,11,12] Lateral and oblique views can usually be taken using portable equipment with the horse standing if sedation has been used. Support the head on a headstand to reduce motion. Dorsoventral views and radiographs of massive-headed horses such as draft horses and some stallions may require a short-acting anesthetic to prevent motion during long exposure times. Oblique radiographs provide distinction between the contralateral arcades and are the best views for tooth root evaluation. Lateral views allow visualization of the paranasal sinuses and can help rule out the presence of fluid or masses in the sinuses. Draining tracts can be followed from outside the mouth using radiopaque contrast media or sterile metal probes.

When fluid or abnormal tissue is seen in the sinuses, it may be necessary to create a trephine opening into the affected area to obtain a fluid sample for cytology and bacterial culture and sensitivity. Performing sinuscopy can help diagnose conditions such as tooth root abscesses, neoplasia, cysts, and primary sinuses. This procedure has been described elsewhere.[13,14]

In some cases, the horse may need to be sent to a referral center to undergo further diagnostics, such as computed tomography. Computed tomography creates sectional views of the selected anatomy and provides excellent visualization of the osseous, dental, and soft-tissue structures of the head. Individual tooth roots, abscesses, cysts, sinus fluid, neoplasia, and fractures can be identified.[15,16,17] In addi-

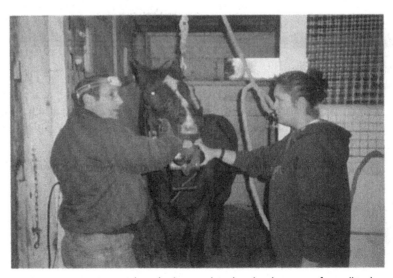

Figure 3.12 Sometimes, suspending the horse's head in the doorway of a stall is the most practical way to support the head.

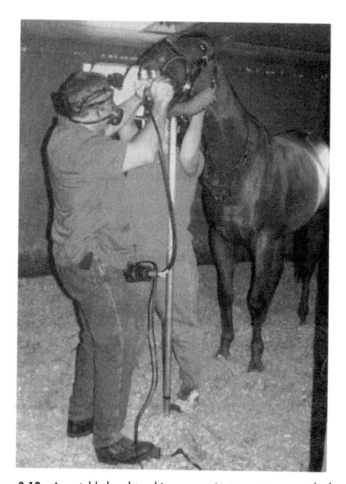

Figure 3.13   A portable headstand is a convenient way to support the head.

tion, three-dimensional reconstructions of the entire head or individual structures can be generated. This diagnostic modality can also be used to further define the nature of abnormalities within the head as well as to establish boundaries for biopsy procedures or surgical exploration (**Table 3.1**).

■ ■   DENTAL CHARTING

Dental charts have many functions. The primary functions are to record observations made during the dental examination, to document procedures performed, and to note future recommendations for treatment. A copy of the chart given to the owner or stable manager lends professionalism and credibility to the dental service

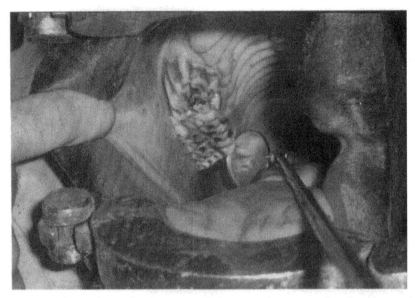

Figure 3.14 Telescoping mechanics' mirrors help in visualizing periodontal pockets and tooth root slivers on the lingual aspects of cheek teeth.

provided. The practitioner has the choice of using available charts or developing his or her own.

A universal system for charting dental abnormalities in the horse is not yet being used. Currently, the Triadan system is recommended for numbering teeth (*Table 3.2*). A system for grading periodontal disease has been adopted from human

TABLE 3.2   Triadan Tooth Numbering System[21-23]

1st number identifies quadrant
The mouth is divided (clockwise from right to left) into 4 quadrants
#100 Upper right quadrant
#200 Upper left quadrant
#300 Lower left quadrant
#400 Lower right quadrant
(Note: The numbers refer to the actual right and left side of the horse.)

2nd number identifies tooth
Central incisor 01
Intermediate incisor 02
Corner incisor 03
Canine 04
Wolf tooth 05
Cheek teeth 06–11

Based on equine dental formula of 44 teeth.
Uses three numbers to identify location of tooth.

TABLE 3.3   **Grades of Periodontal Disease**[20]

+	Local gingivitis with hyperemia and edema
++	Erosion of the gingival margin
+++	Periodontitis with gingival retraction
++++	Gross periodontal pocketing and destruction of alveolar bone

dentistry and is used by some practitioners (*Table 3.3*). Baker has offered a system for grading equine dental caries (*Table 3.4*). *Table 3.5* lists common abbreviations used in charting equine dental abnormalities.

Existing charts are available from the American Association of Equine Practitioners (AAEP) dentistry subcommittee, by Equi-Dent Technologies Inc (www.equi-dent.com), by World Wide Equine Inc, and by the International Association of Equine Dentists (this list is not all-inclusive). A chart can also be computer-generated using Dr. Richard Miller's DataDent software (see following discussion).

The dental chart should contain pertinent details such as contact information for the owner/client, the location of the horse, a brief description of the horse, the condition score of the horse, a brief history of problems that could be related to dental disease, some means of charting out abnormalities and work performed, information on occlusion and lateral excursion, and a section for itemization of services. See *Figure 3.15* for an example of a dental chart designed by Dr. Scott Greene of Equi-Dent Technologies and his suggestions concerning charting.

It is recommended that at least two copies of each chart be generated, by carbon, computer, or copier. In addition to the copy retained by the practitioner, the owner and/or the client or both should receive a copy. Charting each patient enables the practitioner to maintain accurate records while minimizing the chance of forgetting to bill for *all* services performed. The dental chart gives the owner/client a detailed description of the costs of procedures performed, which justifies the total bill. It also emphasizes that equine dentistry is a complex process of analyzing problems and producing and implementing treatment plans.

TABLE 3.4   **Grades of Dental Caries**[20]

Grade 1: Caries of the infundibular cementum
Grade 2: Caries of the infundibular cementum and surrounding
　　　　　 enamel
Grade 3: Caries of the infundibular cementum, enamel, and dentin
Grade 4: Splitting of the tooth as a result of caries
Grade 5: Loss to tooth owing to caries

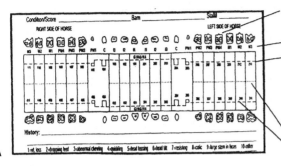

Occlusal diagrams may be used to identify the location of missing or supernumerary teeth, caries, fractures, fragments, diastema as well as teeth that are rotated, misshapen or malaligned.

The classic nomenclature is noted to help practitoners learn the Triadan system.

The Triadan system gives each tooth a number (6's=the 1st cheek teeth or PM-2's) and also indicates in which arcade it is located (206=the left, upper PM-2). The incisors are 1-3, canines are 4's, wolf teeth are 5's and the cheek teeth are 6-11. If you face the horse and raise your left hand, it will be pointing in the direction of the 100 arcade (the horses' right upper arcade). Now proceed in a clock wise fashion around the horses' head to identify the other arcades 200=the horses' upper left, (the practitioners'upper right), 300= lower left, 400=lower right.

Dotted line represents the occlusal surfaces of the upper and lower arcades.

Dashed line denotes the border of the gingiva and the tooth crown.

A

The lined area on 106 indicates the application of bit seats. I apply bit seats on almost all of my patients and I don't note them on my charts. If bit seat application is an elective procedure in your practice, then note them without shading.

The shaded areas designate the location where excessive crown (110) was reduced from the tooth on the opposite side of the line and excessive wear (410) of the tooth possessing the shaded area.

The shaded area on 406 reflects the large hook that was reduced from 106 (prior to bit seat placement) and the wear (and the partial bit seat created by the 106 hook) on 406.

The height of the malocclusions has been noted in millimeters.

The numeric system used in the history and exam section allows for quick, detailed documentation of the abnormalities present and which teeth are involved.

The recommendation section provides an area to document client communications.

The interocclusal space of the cheek teeth is defined as the height of the space between the occlusal surfaces of an opposing pair of teeth or opposing arcades. It is important to record what these measurements are at the completion of the float or prior to and after an incisor reduction.

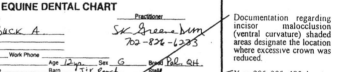

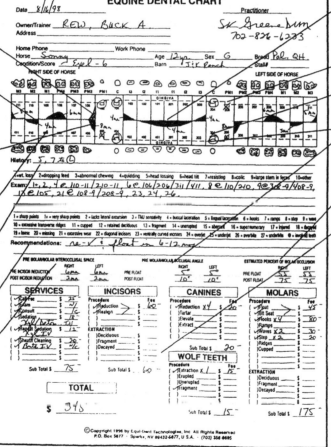

Documentation regarding incisor malocclusion (ventral curvature) shaded areas designate the location where excessive crown was reduced.

X on 205, 305, 405 denotes wolf teeth not present.

O around 104, 105, 204, 304, 404 denotes presence of canines and wolf tooth.

denotes cut and rounded.

The occlusal angle of the cheek teeth is defined as the angle of the chewing surface in relation to a level horizontal line.

The estimated % of molar occlusion is a subjective estimate.

The section for itemization of services provides a detailed description of the cost of the procedure for the client and allows the practitioner a system to maintain consistency in their fee scale.

Fill out a dental chart after each case. This will provide an accurate record and minimize the chance of forgetting to include all services.

Books of 50, 2 part carbonless pages

B

Figure 3.15   A,B. Examples of dental charts designed by Dr. Scott Greene of Equi-Dent Technologies.

TABLE 3.5   Common Dental Abbreviations[19]

SP: sharp enamel points
BI (L, A, or U): buccal injury (laceration, abrasion, ulcer)
LI (L, A, or U): lingual injury (laceration, abrasion, ulcer)
CH: Crown hook
BK: beak
RP: ramp
Sp: step
Wa: wave
ETR: excessive transverse ridges
Cup: cup in central portion of crown
TC: tall crown
PD: periodontal pocket
Fx: fracture
CAL: calculus
DT/R: deciduous root sliver or fragment
CA: cavity
SN: supernumerary tooth
O: missing tooth
WC: worn crown
ROT: rotated
X: extraction

KEY POINT:

The practitioner should inform the owner/client of the work needed and the estimated cost prior to performing any dental services. Only after the practitioner obtains approval to perform the necessary work should any procedures be performed. If possible, require a signature on the chart indicating that the person responsible for the bill was informed of the cost.

At this writing, there is one computer program designed specifically for equine dental practitioners. This program, DataDent, was designed and produced by Richard Miller and computer software engineer Ken Moore. The software can be ordered from Dr. Richard Miller on CD-ROM (Dr. Richard Miller; 13341 Santa Margarita Parkway, Suite A215; Rancho Santa Margarita, CA 92688; 949-858-1975). The program provides the ability to chart procedures, to generate invoices, to perform some bookkeeping procedures, and to sort patients. Digital photographs can be added to patients' charts for more complete documentation. With this program loaded onto your laptop personal computer and connected to a printer, you can provide invoices onsite.

■ ■ REFERENCES

1. Uhlinger C. Survey of selected dental abnormalities in 233 horses. Proceedings for the 33rd Annual Meeting of the American Association of Equine Practitioners 1987;33: 577–583.
2. Kirkland K. A survey of equine dental disease and associated oral pathology. Abstract, Proceedings of the 3rd World Veterinary Dental Congress. Philadelphia, 103.
3. Dixon et al. Equine dental disease, part 1: A long-term study of 400 cases: disorders of incisor, canine and first premolar teeth. Equine Vet J 1999;31(5):369–377.
4. Dixon et al. Equine dental disease, part 2: A long-term study of 400 cases: disorders of development and eruption and variations in the position of cheek teeth. Equine Vet J 1999;31(6):519–528.
5. Dixon et al. Equine dental disease, part 3: A long-term study of 400 cases: disorders of wear, traumatic damage and idiopathic fractures, tumors and miscellaneous disorders of the cheek teeth. Equine Vet J 2000;32(1):9–18.
6. Dixon et al. Equine dental disease, part 4. A long-term study of 400 cases: apical infections of cheek teeth. Equine Vet J 2000;32(3):182–194.
7. Baker GJ. Dental physical examination. In Gaughan EM, DeBowes RM, eds. Veterinary Clinics of North America: Equine Practice. Vol. 14(2), August 1998. Philadelphia: Saunders, 247–257.
8. Baker GJ, Kirkland KD. Sedation for dental prophylaxis in the horse: A comparison between detomidine and xylazine. In Proceedings of the American Association of Equine Practitioners, Lexington, KY, 1995, 40.
9. Wagner AE, Muir WW, Hinchcliff KW. Cardiovascular effects of xylazine and detomidine in horses. Am J Vet Res 1991;52:651.
10. Park RD. Radiographic examination of the equine head. In Honnas CM, Bertone AL, eds. Veterinary Clinics of North America: Equine Practice. Vol. 9(1), April 1993. Philadelphia: Saunders, 49–74.
11. O'Brien RT, Biller DS. Dental imaging. In Gaughan EM, DeBowes RM, eds. Veterinary Clinics of North America: Equine Practice. Dentistry. Vol. 14(2), August 1998. Philadelphia: Saunders, 259–271.
12. Gibbs C. Dental imaging. In Baker GJ, Easley J, eds. Equine Dentistry. Philadelphia: Saunders, 1999: 139–169.
13. Ruggles AJ, Ross MW, Freeman DE. Endoscopic examination of normal paranasal sinuses in horses. Veterinary Surgery 1991;20:418–423.
14. Ruggles AJ, Ross MW, Freeman DE. Endoscopic examination and treatment of paranasal sinuses in 16 horses. Veterinary Surgery 1993;22:508–514.
15. Barbee DD, Allen JR, Gavin PR. Computed tomography in horses. Veterinary Radiology 1987;28:144–151.
16. Barbee DD, Allen JR. Computed tomography in the horse: general principles and clinical applications. Proc Am Assoc Equine Pract 1986;32:483.
17. Dik KJ. Computed tomography of the equine head. Veterinary Radiology and Ultrasound 1994;35:236.
18. Tietje, S, Becker M, Bockenhoff G. Computed tomographic evaluation of head diseases in the horse: fifteen cases. Equine Veterinary Journal 1996;28:98–105.

19. MQ Lowder. Current nomenclature for the equine dental arcade. Veterinary Med 1998;August:754–755.
20. Floyd MR. The modified Triadan system: nomenclature for veterinary dentistry. J Veterinary Dentistry 1991;8(4):18.
21. Foster DL. Nomenclature for equine dental anatomy based on the modified Triadan system. Proceedings from the Annual Meeting of the International Association of Equine Dental Technicians. Detroit, 1993, 35.
23. Baker GJ. A study of equine dental disease. PhD Thesis. University of Glasgow, 78–82.
24. Easley KJ. Dental and oral examination. In: Baker GJ, Easley KJ, eds. Equine Dentistry. Philadelphia: Saunders, 1999.

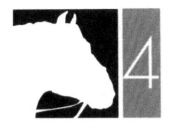

BASIC DENTAL TECHNIQUES

**KRISTIN WILEWSKI, PATRICIA PENCE,
TONY BASILE, AND SCOTT GREEN**

Because horses' teeth continue to erupt, most routine dental procedures for horses involve reducing excess crown. Excess crown is secondary to defects in conformation of the head, to abnormalities in individual teeth, to injury, and to diet. Defects in conformation, such as brachynathism and prognathism, prevent normal incisor wear. Any tooth not opposed by a tooth of equal size will have parts that overgrow because they are not being worn off. Molar tables that are shifted slightly forward or backward of their opposing tables will result in excess crown on the most cranial and/or caudal teeth in the arcade, depending on the type of shift. Abnormal chewing patterns, such as chewing primarily on one side, may prevent adequate wear on the opposite arcade, thus enabling those teeth to grow longer. Chewing in short, up-and-down strokes will create abnormal wear, which manifests as overhanging upper buccal and lower lingual edges or an exaggerated saw-tooth appearance to the occlusal surface.

This chapter will explain how to reduce excess crown in specific areas of the mouth using various instruments. All of the procedures performed on cheek teeth require sedation and use of a full-mouth speculum. Whether to start on the upper or lower arcades is a matter of personal preference. It will save you time, however, if you do your work in the following order:

- reduce long cheek teeth,
- rough out bit seats,
- float the teeth and finish bit seats,

- cut and smooth canines,
- pull wolf teeth, and
- reduce incisors.

What instruments to use depends on personal preference and the instruments available. Always use correct posture, and remember that all instruments are capable of producing severe soft-tissue damage. Be conscious of what your body is doing and what your instruments are doing at all times. When using burrs, always use those with variable speed control.

KEY POINT

▶ Specific types of abnormalities in this book are referred to by the names that are used by equine dentists in the United States at this printing. The names are common and descriptive, not scientific, because no scientific terms have been universally agreed on at this time. Refer to the glossary for definitions of terms used in this book.

PRACTICE TIP

Before doing any work, pick a guide tooth in each arcade. The guide tooth is one that appears to be the appropriate height for that arcade. Use these teeth for reference points when you reduce teeth that are too long. If unsure whether a tooth is too long, examine the tooth in the opposing arcade. It should be shorter than your guide tooth.

■ ■   REDUCING LONG CHEEK TEETH

The Upper Arcades

Excess Crown Appearing as Rostral Hooks or Long #106 and #206. If the rostral portion of #106 or #206 is longer than the caudal portion and narrower than it is wide, the tooth will have a hooked appearance. Extremely long hooks look like fangs. Rostral hooks are most readily recognized when viewed across the tongue looking at the lingual or medial aspect (*Fig. 4.1A, B*).

KEY POINT

▶ The true mass of a hook can more easily be appreciated when viewed from the lingual side of the tooth.

Hand files. Small hooks can be reduced by filing with a short, angled float with a solid carbide blade in the push position. Start by filing the lingual aspect of the rostral surface of the tooth until the lingual part of the hook is reduced. File the buccal

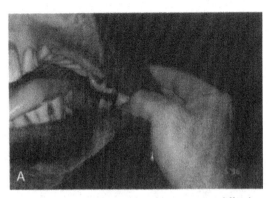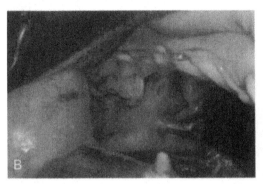

Figure 4.1 **A.** It is more difficult to recognize rostral hooks when viewed from the front or from the buccal aspect. **B.** The bulk of the hook is more apparent when viewed from the lingual aspect.

edge by introducing the float into the interdental space on the side opposite the tooth and filing until the buccal edge is blended with the lingual edge (*Fig. 4.2A–C*). Make sure all overly long areas of the tooth are removed, especially on the buccal side, and reestablish the table angle. Do not simply round off the hook, leaving part of the rostral portion of the tooth longer than the caudal portion.

Reciprocal files. Large or small rostral hooks can also be reduced using an electric or air-driven file. The technique is similar to that used for hand filing. An angled file is used, and the tooth is shaped by filing at various angles and cross floating the same as described for hand filing.

Burrs. Rostral hooks can be reduced by using rotary burrs. Start at the rostral aspect of the tooth and reduce the hook as you move caudally, making sure to not keep the burr in one spot for too long. A small (1/2-inch) round diamond-cut burr works well for small rostral hooks. Larger hooks may need a larger (5/8-inch) round, cylindrical diamond-cut burr, or the conical burr by Equi-Dent. You can switch to the smaller (1/2-inch) burr when finishing the edges near the palate and cheek. The tongue may need to be pulled off to the opposite side by an assistant. Use a forefinger or thumb to push the palate away from the tooth, particularly #206, so that it will not be damaged (*Fig. 4.3A, B*). The direction the burr spins makes it more likely to catch the palate on the horse's left side. Pull the cheek away from the tooth to prevent soft-tissue damage when burring the rostral buccal edge. The caudal buccal edge must be finished by hand after the floating is completed.

KEY POINT
▶ Hold burr handpieces using a pencil-grip, that is, with the index finger extended and guiding the handpiece and the thumb supporting the handpiece on the

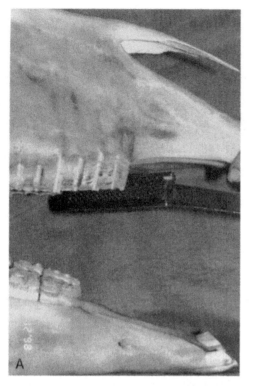

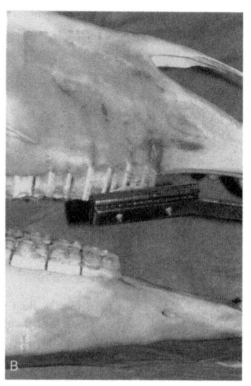

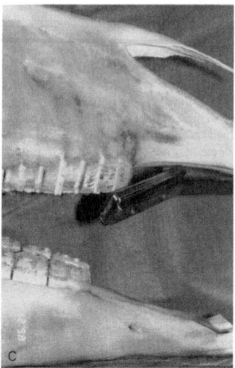

Figure 4.2 Small rostral hooks can be reduced by hand filing the lingual aspect to the rostral surface first (**A**), then filing the buccal edge (**B**), and finally introducing the float blade into the mouth on the side opposite the tooth being floated (**C**), and filing the tooth until the buccal edge is blended with the lingual edge.

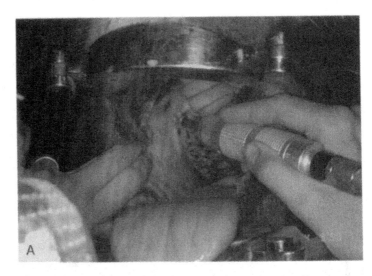

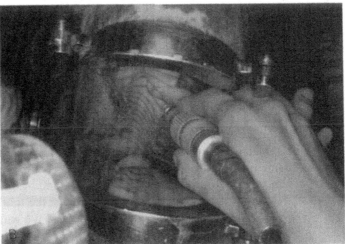

Figure 4.3 **A.** A round burr can be used to reduce small rostral hooks or to create bit seats. The thumb or forefinger is used to push the palate away from the tooth when burring the lingual aspect of #206. **B.** Use the index finger of the opposite hand to push the palate away from the burr when working on the #206 teeth.

opposite side. The remaining fingers should be curled around the handpiece. This grip also applies to handpieces with guards attached.

PRACTICE TIP

Mount each size of your burrs and cutting wheels in its own handpiece. It is faster to pop off a handpiece than it is to change a burr.

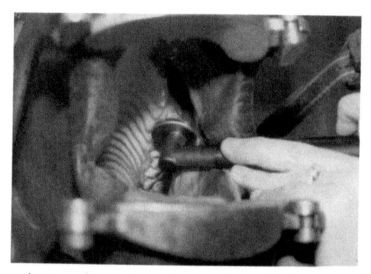

Figure 4.4   The Power Float can be used to remove rostral hooks and create bit seats. (Photograph courtesy of Power Float.)

Rotary files. The rotating disk burrs on Rach's Power Float or the Swissfloat work well on anterior hooks (*Fig. 4.4*). Technique for the Power Float will be described in this chapter. Use this same technique to create bit seats with this instrument. To reduce tooth #206, hold the motor using a pistol-grip perpendicular to the long axis of the horse so the motor is sticking out the left side of the horse's mouth. Hold the right angle portion of the grinding disk with the thumb and forefinger of your left hand to steady the instrument. You can stabilize the head of the float with your hand either inside the mouth or outside of it, depending on the size of your hand and what feels comfortable to you. Reduce and shape the tooth with the grinding disk. You can slide obliquely across the mouth to the #106 with the motor still in your right hand.

PRACTICE TIP

Use some type of water cooling system to keep the tooth from overheating when working on large hooks or ramps.

Molar cutters. Simple or compound action D-head cutters may be used to reduce long #106 and #206 hooks (*Fig. 4.5*). The width of the hook will determine the type of cutter needed.

Equi-Chip. Small hooks can also be quickly removed by using an Equi-Chip (*Fig. 4.6A, B*). Insert a wedge gag to hold the mouth open. Place the Equi-Chip with the

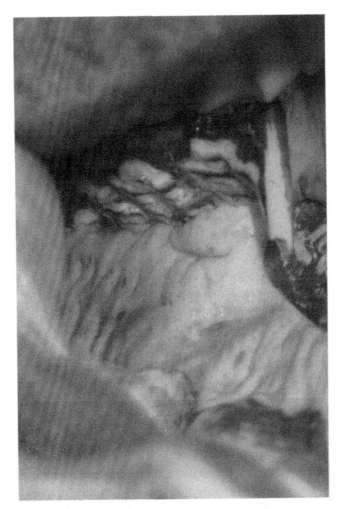

Figure 4.5 A hook of this size should be first reduced with molar cutters. This hook was wide enough at the base to require D-head compound cutters.

blade pulled back toward you on the rostral aspect of the hook with the handle raised up so that the instrument will cut at a downward angle. An assistant then pushes the handle in a quick, firm motion, shearing off the hook. This instrument is not precise, and too little or too much tooth may be removed. As with all cutters, the tooth must be reshaped and smoothed by filing or burring after being cut. Again, be sure all the overlong tooth is removed and that the table angle is reestablished. This method is not recommended for geriatric horses because the entire tooth may be knocked out.

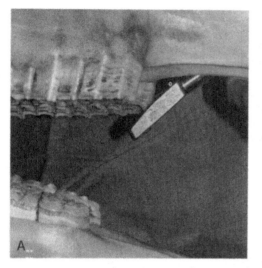
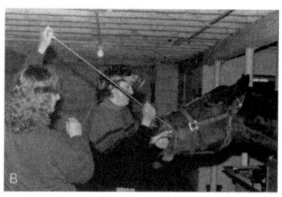

Figure 4.6 A. When using the Equi-Chip to remove rostral hooks on #106 and #206, the cutting blade must be positioned on the rostral aspect of the hook. **B.** Raise the handle until it is at approximately a 45–65° angle above the tooth. Slide the sliding handle firmly into the cutter in one smooth motion.

PRACTICE TIP

When using the Equi-Chip to cut a rostral hook, filing a notch on the front of the tooth where you want the blade to cut will help make the cut more precise.

Excess Crown in #107–110 and #207–210

Hand files. If these teeth are slightly long, they can be reduced by filing the occlusal surface with a coarse solid carbide or Capps blade in the push configuration. Use a float with a short obtuse handle for the #7s and a long obtuse handle for the #8–10s. Use one hand to operate the file and the other hand inside the mouth to guide the file. File the lingual aspect at this time. The buccal side will be filed when you float. Be sure to maintain the occlusal table angle.

Reciprocating files. Reciprocating files can be used to reduce moderate or severely long teeth. Use the long offset handle and the file in the push position (*Fig. 4.7*).

Burrs. Long upper cheek teeth can be reduced using an extended burr with a low-profile guard (Harlan or Carbide Products). The low-profile guard allows more of the burr to be exposed for greater visibility and better access to the tooth surface. Introduce the burr over the top of the tongue or straight in alongside the tongue. Work the burr over the surface of the long tooth until it is level with the rest of the arcade. Round off the lingual edge and restore the table angle.

Rotary files. Rotary files can be used to reduce these teeth. Do not work on one tooth too long, or you will overheat it. Work obliquely across the mouth instead of parallel with the teeth. Hold the pistol grip in one hand and the shaft of the float with the thumb and index finger of the other hand, as you would hold a pool cue. Rest the back of that hand lightly at the intersection of the incisor plate and the shafts of the speculum to stabilize the float. You may wish to hold the speculum with the remaining fingers of that hand.

Tilt the grinding surface slightly so that the right angle of the float is pressing against the buccal mucosa. Pressure from the cheeks helps support the instrument. Appropriate positioning of the guard and the right angle of the float head will prevent lingual and buccal abrasion.

Molar cutters. An upper tooth that is erupting into the space of a missing lower tooth can be reduced with molar cutters after the rest of the arcade has been corrected and floated. Usually, a compound action D-head cutter will be needed (*Fig. 4.8*). Have an assistant pull the tongue to the opposite side. Introduce the cutter into the mouth until it hits the long tooth. Open the jaws and seat the blade. Position the handles level with the arcade. Once positioning is verified, close the handles and shear the tooth. Reestablish the table angle, and smooth any sharp edges with hand files or a burr.

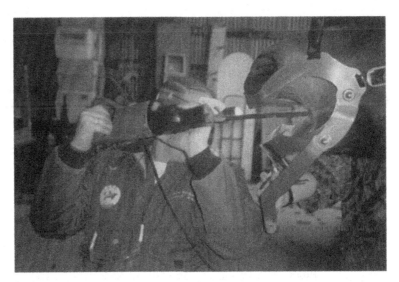

Figure 4.7 Reciprocating file on upper cheek teeth. Turn the whole instrument upside down when using the long, straight float handle on the upper arcades. That way, you can quickly turn it over to work on the lower arcades without removing the handle. Insert the offset float handles upside down with the motor right side up. This is more comfortable. (Equipment by Equi-Dent Technologies.)

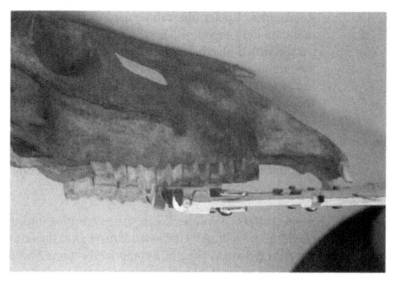

Figure 4.8 Cutting maxillary teeth requires a compound-action D-head molar cutter. (Photograph courtesy of World Wide Equine.)

Excess Crown in #111 and #211

KEY POINT
▶ In addition to excess crown, the upper #11s may have sharp enamel points that protrude into the cheeks. It is not unusual to discover abrasions or lacerations in the mucosa over these teeth.

Hand files. World Wide Equine makes a low-profile, long-handled file with a solid carbide blade mounted on it at an angle that works well for small hooks. Capps makes a similar float that cuts very aggressively. With either float, position the head behind the tooth and pull toward you using short strokes.

Reciprocating files. Owing to the proximity of the mandibular bone and soft tissue, there is a greater chance of causing damage to these areas with a reciprocating unit. Do not use a reciprocating file on these hooks until you are very comfortable using it and are familiar with how far back the caudal stroke goes. Use a long-handled file with a 30° pull cut blade. If you can, guide the file with one hand inside the mouth.

Burrs. Hooks and accentuated transverse ridges can be reduced using a 6–10 inch burr (Carbide Products, Harlton) with a guard. Equi-Dent offers an instrument called the caudal hook grinder that is designed specifically for use on these abnormalities (*Fig. 4.9*). When using Harlton's burrs, use the high-profile guard because it provides extra protection for the soft palate. Because there is not much room to

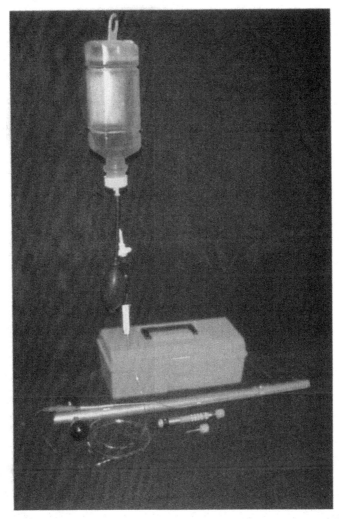

Figure 4.9 The caudal hook grinder manufactured by Equi-Dent allows excellent visibility while reducing hooks on the #11 teeth. Attach a bottle of water as shown to cool the tooth being worked on. (Photograph courtesy of Equi-Dent Technologies.)

work in this area, be careful the horse does not chew on the burr. Introduce the burr as previously described, and work it over the surface of the long tooth until it is level with the rest of the arcade. Restore the table angle, and finish the caudal, lingual, and buccal edges with a large S file.

Rotary floats. Rach's Power Float can be used on these hooks (*Fig. 4.10*). The head of the Swissfloat may be too large to fit in the buccal pocket. The technique is the same as for the #08, #09, and #10 teeth. Beware of grinding the gingiva in the Curve of Spee.

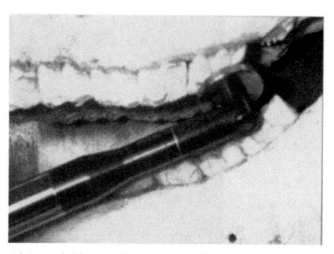

Figure 4.10 The guarded low-profile rotary head of the Power Float can fit into the buccal space of most horses to reduce sharp points on the caudal maxillary teeth of the upper arcades.

Equi-Chip. Small hooks can be quickly reduced using the Equi-Chip. Place the blade behind the hook and hold it in place while an assistant pulls the slide out with a snapping motion (*Fig. 4.11A, B*). A large S file can be used to smooth off any rough edges.

Molar cutters. Large hooks can be cut off with molar cutters, but care must be taken to avoid soft-tissue damage. Use a simple D-head cutter if you are only cutting off a

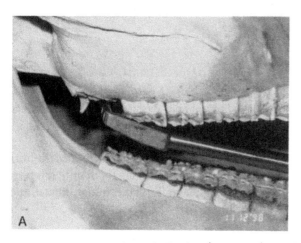
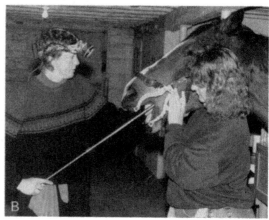

Figure 4.11 **A.** When using the Equi-Chip to remove caudal #11 hooks, position the blade on the caudal aspect of the hook. **B.** Pull the sliding handle out in one smooth, swift motion until the cutter delivers a cutting blow to the hook. The handle needs to be nearly parallel to the lower arcades to cut an upper #11 hook.

hook. If the whole tooth is long, you will need a compound-action D-head cutter. Correct and float the rest of the arcade first. Position the cutter blades on the tooth, hold the handles level with the arcade, and cut the tooth. Reestablish the table angle, and burr or file any sharp edges.

KEY POINT

▶ The caudal cheek teeth are closest to the physiological hinge (the TM joint). Leaving any of these teeth too long will subject them to tremendous pressure. The result will be pain during mastication and an imbalanced mouth. Remove the speculum and check lateral excursion and carefully compare the grinding sound of the caudal cheek teeth with the rostral cheek teeth. If the caudal cheek teeth feel uneven or sound louder, or if there is no grinding sound at all coming from the rostral cheek teeth, put the speculum back in and carefully inspect the teeth to be sure they are level, balanced, and have the table angle restored.

Lower Arcades

Excess Crown Appearing as Rostral Ramps in #306 and #406

Hand files. Teeth #306 and #406, if long, tend to be tallest at the rostral tip sloping down in a "ramp"-like fashion caudally. This abnormality is commonly referred to as a ramp because it is wider than it is long. Use a short, straight float with a solid carbide blade or a Capps blade in the push position. Position the horse's head just below eye level. Place the float on the teeth caudal to the #6 and pull forward. It helps if you use your opposite hand to guide the float and apply slight pressure as you pull over the ramp itself. File the tooth, restoring the table angle as you file, until it is level with the rest of the arcade.

Reciprocating files. Even pronounced ramps can be corrected quickly with a reciprocating float. Use a straight-handled file, and restore the table angle as the tooth is reduced.

Burrs. Use a carbide chip drum burr (Equi-Dent), 4-inch burr with burr guard (the high-profile guard if using Harlton's). Have an assistant hold the tongue to the opposite side. Ensure the guard is placed between the tongue and the burr because the direction the burr spins in makes it easy to catch the tongue if it is not properly protected. Pull the cheek away from the burr with the fingers of your opposite hand, or use a buccal guard (Equi-Dent or other) to protect the cheek. If using a burr with a guard, position the guard to protect the gingival tissue and tongue. The technique is reversed for #406. Finally, restore the table angle.

Rotary burrs. Use the same technique as for #106 and #206. Use your thumb to push the loose gingival tissue out of the way.

Molar cutters. An extremely long #306 or #406 can be reduced by cutting with the proper size simple joint cutter. The C-head cutter is usually the correct size, but individual cases vary. Be aware that owing to the shape of these teeth (narrow rostrally), the cutters may slide off the tooth rostrally, or the tooth may fracture with the rostral aspect shorter than the caudal part. After you cut the tooth, restore the table angle by burring or filing.

Excess Crown in #307–310 and #407–410

Hand files. The most common long teeth in this group are #308, #309, #408, and #409. If these teeth are only slightly long, they can be reduced by hand filing using a long, straight float with an aggressive solid carbide or Capps blade (*Fig. 4.12*). Restore the table angle as the teeth are reduced.

Reciprocating file. A reciprocating file can be used to reduce these teeth and reestablish the table angle quickly and effortlessly. Use the long, straight handle (*Fig. 4.13*). The buccal edges of the arcade can also be rounded off at this time.

Burrs. A 6-inch extended burr with a guard (the high-profile guard if using Harlton's) is best to work on these teeth because the 4-inch guard is too short to reach tooth #09. Have an assistant pull the tongue to the opposite side, and introduce the burr, using the guard to protect the base of the tongue. The tongue can easily become caught in the burr if it is not shielded. Reduce the teeth by moving the burr in sweeping lingual-buccal motions. Push the guard as close to the cheek as possible to prevent creating a ridge on the buccal aspect of the teeth. When finished, the teeth should be level with the rest of the arcade, the buccal edge rounded off, and the table angle restored.

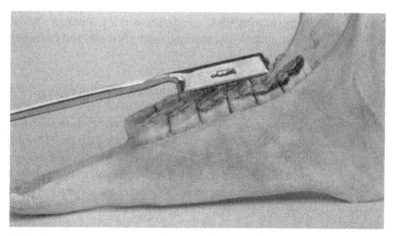

Figure 4.12 The aggressive cutting surface of the Capps float blades makes it possible to reduce small to medium waves by hand. (Photograph courtesy of World Wide Equine.)

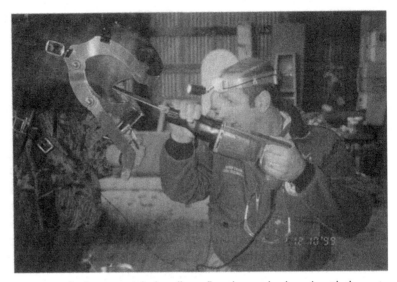

Figure 4.13 Use the long, straight handle to float lower cheek teeth with the reciprocating float.

Molar cutters. If these teeth are extremely long, simple or compound joint molar cutters can quickly reduce them to level (*Fig. 4.14*). The D-head cutter is usually the proper size, but some may be narrow enough to require the C-head cutter. Keep the handles level with the arcade, and make your cuts from rostral to caudal. After cutting, reestablish the table angle and round the buccal edges by burring or filing.

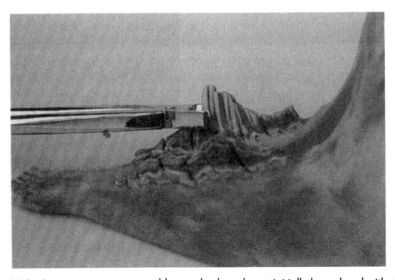

Figure 4.14 Severe waves or stepped lower cheek teeth can initially be reduced with simple-action D-head molar cutters.

Excess Crown Appearing as Caudal Hooks or Long #311 and #411

KEY POINT

▶ It is important to be able to distinguish #311 and #411 teeth that are truly long or hooked from those that are tipped up caudally because they are within the Curve of Spee. *Figs. 1.xx* in Chapter 1 illustrate this difference.

Horses with short heads, such as Arabians and ponies, tend to have the #11s in this curve, creating the illusion that they are pathologically long. An easy way to tell the difference is by palpating the lower #11 and comparing it with the opposing upper #11. If they are protruding equal distances from the gingival margin, then the lower #11 is the appropriate length and the horse just has a crowded mandible. If the lower #11 protrudes further than the upper, then it is too long and must be reduced.

It is not unusual to see hooks on the lower #11 if the upper #6s have hooks because the entire upper arcade is shifted slightly forward, leaving the caudal aspect of the lower #11 with no opposing occlusal surface to grind against.

Hand files. Small hooks and accentuated transverse ridges on #311 and #411 can be reduced by filing with a long, straight float with an aggressive solid carbide or Capps blade set in the pull position. Use short strokes to minimize damage to the mucosa caudal to the tooth.

Reciprocating files. Because of the close proximity of soft tissue and bone, reciprocating files should be used with utmost caution, if used at all. Use a reciprocating file only if you are very comfortable with the placement of the caudal part of the stroke. Use a long, straight file and be very careful. If possible, keep one hand inside the mouth to guide the file. Restore the table angle as the tooth is reduced.

Burrs. Moderate hooks or moderately long lower #11s can be reduced most easily by burring. If you are using Harlton's equipment, use the 6-inch extended burr with the high-profile guard. Carbide products makes 8-inch and 10-inch burrs with guards that make working on this tooth easier if the horse has a large head (*Fig. 4.15*). Equi-Dent's caudal hook grinder works well because its diameter is small enough to allow adequate visualization of the tooth while you are working on it. This unit uses a carbide chip burr, which is less aggressive and causes less tissue damage.

Rotary files. The Swiss Float or Rach's Power Float can also be applied to reducing these teeth.

Molar cutters. Moderate to large hooks or excessively long #11s can be reduced with molar cutters. Most hooks can be cut with a B-head or C-head simple joint cutter, but the occasional large hook may require a simple D-head cutter. Correct the

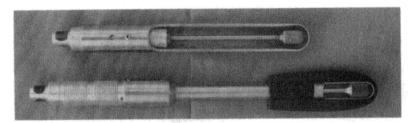

Figure 4.15 Low-profile burr guards allow work on upper and lower caudal molars. Shown are Harlan's stainless steel guard for the 8-inch burr (*top*) and the plastic guard for the 12-inch burr by Carbide Products (*bottom*).

rest of the arcade before attempting to cut the tooth. Have an assistant pull the tongue out to the opposite side to prevent it being caught in the cutter. Slide the cutter over the teeth rostral to the tooth being cut until you reach the #11. Open and position the cutter on the tooth, keeping the handles level with the arcade (*Fig. 4.16A, B*). After positioning has been rechecked, close the cutter without moving the handles out of position. Positioning the molar cutters on the lower #11s is more critical than any other tooth because if the handles are lifted up, the blades tilt down and can cut into the mandible itself. After cutting, smooth the tooth and restore the table angle with a file or burr.

FLOATING

The goal of floating is to remove sharp points and round the upper buccal and lower lingual edges of the teeth. When finished, these edges should be rounded and smooth (*Fig. 4.17A–E*). Proper floating reduces discomfort caused by sharp edges when the horse is chewing and when bridled with a tight cavesson. Floating is finished with hand files or reciprocating files. Regardless of which instrument is used, the blades are in the same push setting or pull setting, and the shape of handle used, whether straight or angled, is the same in each area of the mouth.

The upper cheek teeth can be floated without using a full-mouth speculum (*Fig. 4.18A, B*). Do not let the horse chew on the float blades. This can be prevented by not floating too far mesially onto the occlusal surface. Put the full-mouth speculum back in to evaluate your work and to perform finish work, blending the buccal edge with the occlusal surface.

The Upper Arcades

The premolars are floated using a short, angled float with either a carbide chip blade or a solid carbide blade. If a solid carbide blade is used, it should be set in the push configuration. The right hand is used to float the horse's left arcade, and the left

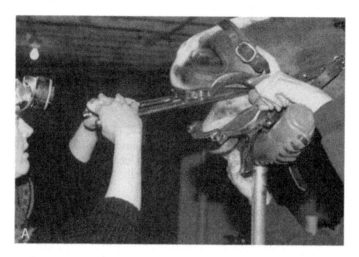

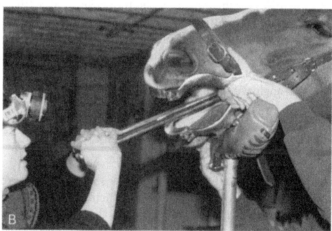

Figure 4.16 **A.** Improper position of handles of molar cutters. Do not raise the handles when cutting caudal mandibular cheek teeth. **B.** Proper position. The handles of the molar cutters should be parallel to the occlusal surface. Have an assistant pull the tongue to one side so it does not get cut.

hand is used to float the right arcade. The teeth should be rounded starting at the ventral aspect of the buccal enamel point. After the sharp edge is removed, float dorsally from that point up the buccal side of the tooth. Blend the floating into the chewing surface. The blended area should feel smooth and curved without defined corners or flat spots.

KEY POINT
▶ Performance horses should have extra floating performed on the buccal ridges of the premolars to maximize comfort, especially when a tight cavesson is used (*Fig. 4.19*).

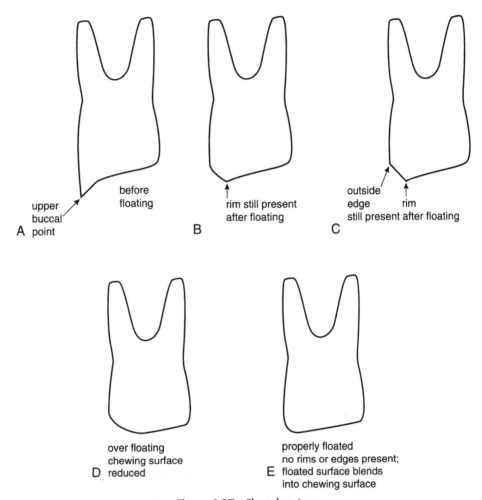

Figure 4.17 Float drawings.

The molars are floated using either a long, straight float handle with a regular-sized blade or a long, angled float with a short float blade. If a solid carbide blade is used, it should be set in the pull configuration. The molars are floated from caudal to rostral as above, starting from the bottom of the buccal points, moving up the buccal side of the tooth. Use a long, angled float to smooth the caudal buccal corners of the #11s.

The Lower Arcades

The premolars and molars are floated in the same fashion in the lower arcades. Put in a full-mouth speculum, and position the horse's head at a level that is comfortable for you. Float the horse's left arcade with your right hand and the right arcade

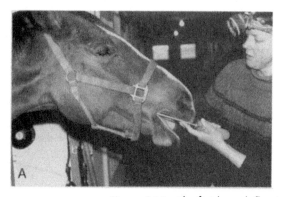
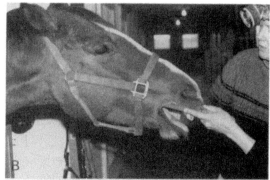

Figure 4.18   The finish work floating on upper cheek teeth can be done without a speculum. Using flat float handles makes it easier to visualize the position of the blade when no speculum is in place. **A.** Start by floating off the bottom of the buccal point. **B.** Next, float the upper buccal surface to reduce vertical enamel folds.

with your left hand. Pull the tongue out of the way with the opposite hand, or have your assistant help you.

The lingual side is floated and rounded by first using a long, straight-handled float with an aggressive carbide blade set in the pull configuration. Use this blade to remove the lingual enamel points. Next, use a float with an offset handle to finish

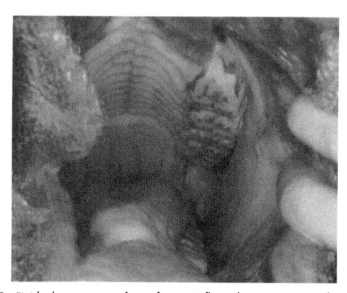

Figure 4.19   Finished appearance of a performance float. There are no upper buccal or lower lingual points or enamel rims. The vertical enamel ridges on the buccal surfaces are reduced. The cheek teeth and incisors are of equal height. There is a 10–15° table angle on the occlusal surfaces. The corners of the rostral cheek teeth are rounded and blended into the other surfaces.

rounding the lingual edges, paying special attention to the #9s and #10s. These teeth are often slightly shorter than the rest of the teeth in the arcade; therefore, use the toe of this float to round the lingual edge.

Use a full-mouth speculum to perform a final examination of your floating. Often, the final check will reveal sharp points that were missed in the caudal areas of the mouth. Use a long, straight file with a medium to fine blade or a large S file on the lower teeth. For roughness on the caudal corners of the #11s, use the inside curve of a large S file, taking short pulling or rubbing strokes. Smooth off any remaining enamel edge (sometimes called a "rim") on the rest of the upper arcade with the outside curve of the S file, and blend the buccal surface with the occlusal surface. Either a small S file or a round burr on a motorized instrument can be used to finish the rostral corners of the upper and lower #6s.

PRACTICE TIP

Frequently rinsing the tooth dust out of the mouth will allow better visualization of your progress and will help keep the horse's tongue from getting too dry.

Bit Seats

The term "bit seats" refers to the rounded and carefully smoothed rostral corners of the upper and lower #6s (*Fig. 4.20A, B*). Bit seats should be created for any horse that carries a bit in its mouth, especially performance horses and horses ridden by inex-

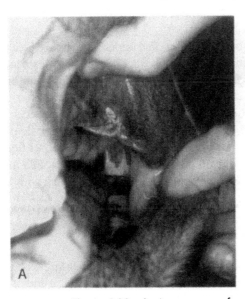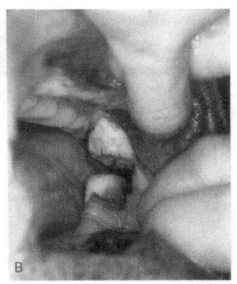

Figure 4.20 A. Appearance of rostral cheek teeth before bit seats are created. **B.** After bit seats are created, the rostral corners are rounded.

perienced riders. There is a varying amount of loose gingival tissue associated with the lower interdental space (the bars). This tissue lies between the bit and the rostral corners of the first cheek teeth and can be sharply pinched if these corners are not rounded off.

Bit seats are performance-enhancing aids for show and work horses because they prevent the horse from being suddenly distracted by pinching of the gums. In horses ridden by inexperienced riders, bit seats can prevent accidents caused by the rider pulling on the reins roughly or inappropriately. Severe, unexpected pain can cause a horse to react by jumping sideways, rearing, or even falling over backwards.

The easy way to create bit seats is by using a 1/2-inch round burr or a bit seat burr (made by Equi-Dent) on a motorized instrument with a flexible shaft (see *Fig. 4.3A, B*). Put in a full-mouth speculum, and position the horse's head at eye level. Have an assistant pull the tongue out of the way. Use your free hand or a buccal cheek retractor to pull the cheek out of the way when shaping the buccal side of the tooth. When shaping the lingual side of #206, push the palate out of the way with a finger because the burr spins into the palate on this side. Shape #106 and #206 until the rostral aspect of the occlusal surface and the rostral edge are blended into a gentle curve that terminates at the gingival margin. Similarly, create bit seats in #306 and #406, being careful to guard the tongue and buccal mucosa. Use a light touch and short strokes. Do not leave the burr in one place too long, or you will burr out a pit in the tooth.

When you are finished, the corner of the tooth should resemble the shape of the tip of a finger and be just as smooth. The amount of tooth removed depends on your preference and experience, but do not remove more than one-quarter of the occlusal surface.

Bit seats can also be created by hand filing. The upper bit seats are filed using an upper premolar float. Start by filing the lingual aspect of the rostral surface of the upper #6s until it is filed to the gingival margin. The buccal edge is then finished by cross-filing (introducing the float into the interdental space on the opposite side of the tooth) and filing until the buccal edge is blended with the lingual edge. A small S file can be used to finish any rough edges and completely blend the floating until no edges remain. The lower bit seats are created using the lower offset float with a carbide blade in the push configuration, keeping the handle down. File the rostral aspects of the lower #6s at various angles until rounded, then finish with a small S file until no edges remain.

Canine Teeth

Canine teeth of male horses usually grow to be long and sharp. Mares can also have canine teeth, but they are tiny, usually appear only in the mandibles, and usually appear during middle-age. Canine teeth are designed to be used for self-defense by stallions protecting their band of mares and are obviously of no use for saddle

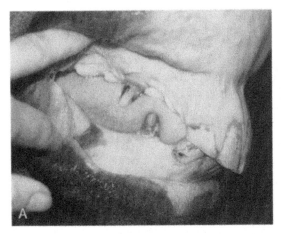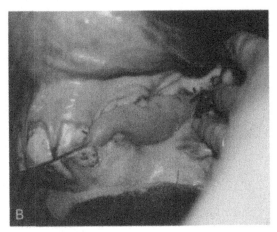

Figure 4.21   **A.** Mature canine teeth are long and sharp before reduction. **B.** After reduction and smoothing off sharp edges.

horses. Canines can get caught on fences and gates, they can catch the bit or the handler's hand as the horse is bridled and unbridled, pinch or lacerate the tongue, cause deep gouges in the flesh of other horses, and interfere with dental procedures. The solution is to cut, file, or burr them off just above the gingival margin (*Fig. 4.21A, B*). The pulp is entered only rarely and can be cauterized with silver nitrate sticks if necessary. After reducing the height of the canine, smooth the remaining tooth into a curved surface.

Sometimes canine teeth fail to erupt and cause discomfort to the horse. This condition can occur in both male and female horses. The owner of the horse usually complains that suddenly the horse resents either taking the bit or having it removed. Unerupted canines appear as a spot of blanched white or red inflamed gingiva caudal to the corner incisors. Palpating the area may be painful to the horse.

Exposing the tip of the canine will speed eruption. Incise and remove a small piece of the mucosa over the tooth by grasping it with a pair of hemostats and snipping it off with sharp surgical scissors or a scalpel blade (*Fig. 4.22*). If the canine is not ready to erupt, the incision will heal over.

Wolf Tooth Extraction

The first premolars, the #5s, are commonly called wolf teeth. These small, vestigial structures may have been a functional part of the arcade millions of years ago. A horse may have just one wolf tooth, both upper wolf teeth, upper and lower wolf teeth, abnormally positioned wolf teeth, unerupted wolf teeth, any combination of these, or no wolf teeth at all. Wolf teeth are removed in horses that have to carry a bit for the same reason that the rostral corners of the second premolars are fashioned

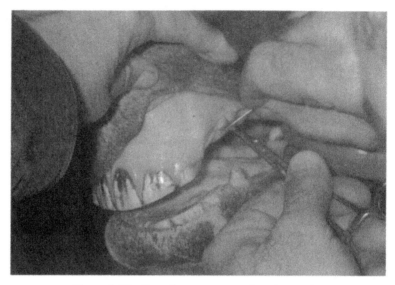

Figure 4.22   Exposing an unerupted canine tooth.

into bit seats—to prevent discomfort to the horse from the redundant tissue on the lower jaws being pinched between the teeth and the bit. It is not necessary to remove wolf teeth in brood mares and stallions that are not ridden.

Prior to removing wolf teeth, sedate the horse and pretreat for postoperative pain. Whether or not to use a local anesthetic depends on the preference of the practitioner, the anticipated difficulty of extraction, and the temperament of the horse. If a local anesthetic is to be given, infiltrate the gingiva surrounding the wolf tooth with 2% lidocaine using a 5/8-inch 25-gauge needle. Approximately 1 cc per tooth should be sufficient.

A full-mouth speculum may hinder the approach to the wolf teeth, so its use is optional. Position the horse's head so that the wolf teeth are at or just below eye level. Which wolf tooth elevator to use is a matter of personal preference, but try to use the smallest one needed to prevent excess soft-tissue damage.

Elevate the mucosa with a half-moon, Burgess, or smaller elevator completely around the tooth before attempting extraction. Elevate the rostral, lingual, and buccal aspects of the tooth. Then position the elevator between the wolf tooth and the #6 tooth caudal to it (*Fig. 4.23*). Push the elevator deep along the caudal part of the root, rocking it gently as you push. Do not use the #6 tooth as a fulcrum, or you will be more likely to break off the root. Elevate the root out of the alveolus. You may have to work deeper on another side of the tooth to break all the periodontal attachments. Try to avoid breaking off the root. Cut any gingival attachments with the elevator, scissors, or a scalpel before you pull out the entire tooth. There will be copious dripping of blood from the surgery site for a few minutes. Remove the tooth with wolf tooth or another type of forceps.

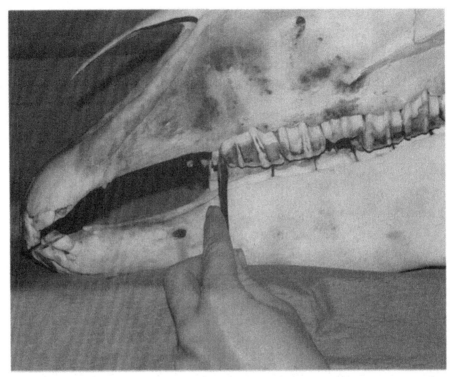

Figure 4.23 Normally positioned wolf teeth. Position the half-moon elevator between the caudal aspect of the wolf tooth and the rostral aspect of the first cheek tooth.

KEY POINT

▶ If the root of the wolf tooth breaks during extraction and cannot be easily re-moved with forceps, don't traumatize the bone by looking for it. Unextracted wolf tooth roots either erupt to the surface on their own or fuse into the alveo-lus. They rarely cause problems. Check the extraction site in 30–60 days. The fragment may work its way to the surface, where it can be removed. Sometimes they do not appear for some time, making it seem as though the horse has grown a new wolf tooth.

Warning: Blood streaming from the surgery site under pressure is a sign that the palatine artery has been punctured. This is of serious concern, so all further dental procedures on this horse must cease for the day, and first aid to control the bleeding must be initiated. A pressure bandage can be applied by putting a clean, rolled-up terry cloth towel (or other soft, absorbent cloth) into the mouth against the punc-ture and tying the mouth closed with brown gauze or tape. For sufficient pressure to be applied, the cloth needs to be bulky enough that it is slightly difficult to close the mouth. The horse should be kept sedated until the bleeding is under control.

Occasionally, wolf teeth erupt lingual to the rostral aspect of #106 or #206. Lingually displaced wolf teeth are often too close to these premolars to get an elevator in between them. One way to extract these teeth is to place an osteotome between the wolf tooth and the #6 tooth, parallel to the tooth, holding it there while an assistant firmly taps the osteotome with a hammer until the wolf tooth is loose. Brace the osteotome to prevent it from slipping lingually. Dissect the tooth from the gingiva, and remove with forceps or fingers.

Wolf teeth found unerupted rostral to the #6 teeth are commonly referred to as blind wolf teeth. They erupt out of the bone but not through the skin and are often found protruding on the buccal aspect of the interdental space. These teeth can be especially uncomfortable when the horse is carrying a bit.

Infiltrate the gingiva over the tooth with 1 mL 2% lidocaine. Sharply incise over the tooth. Introduce a wolf tooth elevator or osteotome at the rostral aspect of the tooth, and work it under the tooth caudally until the tooth is loose. This usually requires the elevator or osteotome to be worked in a parallel rather than perpendicular manner against the bone because the tooth lies parallel to it. Sometimes the elevating instrument must be tapped with a hammer to loosen the tooth, so brace it to prevent it from slipping. Extract the tooth with fingers or forceps, and smooth any rough edges of bone with a bone rasp or rongeurs. The incision is left open to heal.

Lower wolf teeth that are blind or impacted should be removed during the off-season for a performance horse because it may take 1–2 months before the horse can comfortably carry a bit again. The extraction sites for lower wolf teeth cannot drain, so the wound should be flushed daily with a mild antibacterial solution. Healing will be enhanced if the surgery is performed as atraumatically as possible and if the wounds are cleaned and flushed daily until closed. Complications secondary to poor wound drainage and excessive mandibular bone trauma include osteomyelitis and bone spur formation.

Incisor Procedures

Adequate occlusion of the cheek teeth is controlled to a great extent by the conformation of the incisors. When the incisors are too long, there are only two points of contact between the upper and lower jaws: the temporomandibular joint caudally and the incisors rostrally. Contact between the upper and lower incisors is not continuous during mastication when incisors are uneven in length. The mouth has to be opened for the mandible to move, which causes abnormal chewing patterns. The final result is abnormal wear on the cheek teeth.

The goal of incisor bite realignment is to allow good occlusion of the cheek teeth. Most horses will be in good molar occlusion when there is 5 mm or less slide by the incisors before the cheek teeth make occlusal contact when the mandibles are moved side to side. Not all horses need this procedure, but horses that do will benefit greatly.

Horses maintained in a confinement situation, especially those that eat high-concentrate diets, may not receive enough wear on the incisors to maintain good molar occlusion.

The cheek teeth must be level and floated before reducing the incisors for two reasons: 1) so that an accurate estimate of the amount of incisor reduction can be made, or 2) when there are high spots on the cheek teeth, there will be increased pressure on those high cheek teeth, which will cause discomfort and will interfere with mastication after the incisors are reduced.

Incisor reduction may be contraindicated if compromised molars are present because the increased pressure on these teeth will cause discomfort. This will be discussed in further detail in Chapter 7, "Geriatric Horse Dentistry." For the following description of incisor reduction, it is assumed that the cheek teeth have been properly leveled and floated and that no compromised molars are present.

Minor Incisor Realignment. Incisor realignment procedures can be loosely categorized into two groups depending on the amount of tooth needing removal and the degree of difficulty of the work. Minor incisor realignment is needed when examination reveals that the incisors are straight and relatively even in length and a small gap exists between the cheek teeth.

If the horse has well-balanced incisors that are simply overlong, an equal amount of tooth is reduced from all teeth. A minor realignment may also be used to realign incisors that have erupted unequally, but are not extremely overlong. In this case, most of the filing or burring needs to be done on the overlong teeth to bring them into level alignment with the adjacent incisors.

Some 1, 2, or 3 year olds may not come into complete molar occlusion after reducing the incisors all the way to the gingiva. These young horses that have very short incisors and no evidence of TMJ pain usually maintain weight despite a tiny occlusal gap as evidenced by an 8–10 mm incisor slide.

As with other dental procedures, there is more than one way to reduce incisors.

KEY POINT
▶ Very young horses and horses that graze all day may need only minor incisor work.

Hand filing. An incisor rasp can be used to remove a small amount of tooth (*Fig. 4.24*). Use short strokes to minimize injury to the rostral palate.

Burrs. A minor alignment can also be created using a 5/8-inch cylindrical burr or a carbide chip drum burr. The thumb of the free hand is used to hold the palate away from the burr.

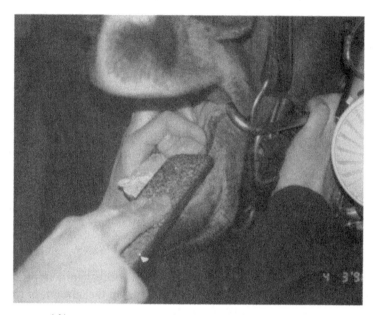

Figure 4.24   Hand filing incisors. Use a wide, flat carbide chip file. Hold the tongue out of the way with the opposite hand when a wedge speculum is in place as it is in this horse.

Major Incisor Realignment.   Horses that need major incisor reduction are those that have greater than 5-mm slide in both directions (*Fig. 4.25A–E*), those with a gap visible between the upper and lower cheek teeth on one or both sides, those in which the incisors are so uneven that the horse lateral excursion of the mandible is inhibited, those with missing incisors or supernumerary incisors, and those with prognathism or brachygnathias.

KEY POINT

▶ Geriatric horses may not need incisor reduction. Those that do must be examined for the presence of compromised cheek teeth before proceeding.

Before proceeding to reduce the incisors, you must evaluate how much incisor needs to be removed and whether all of the incisors are balanced, i.e., of equal length relative to the rest of the teeth in that arcade. The horse's head must be at your eye level to prevent visual distortion of length. Put the incisors into the neutral position by lining up the two center upper teeth with the two center lower teeth. Examine all the incisors from directly in front of the horse and from each side to see if an imaginary line between the upper and lower teeth is straight and level. If this line is not straight and level, determine whether the line is slanted to one side or the other, broken and even, or curves excessively ventrally or dorsally. Next, pull aside each cheek at the commissure, and shine a light on the area where the upper and lower arcades

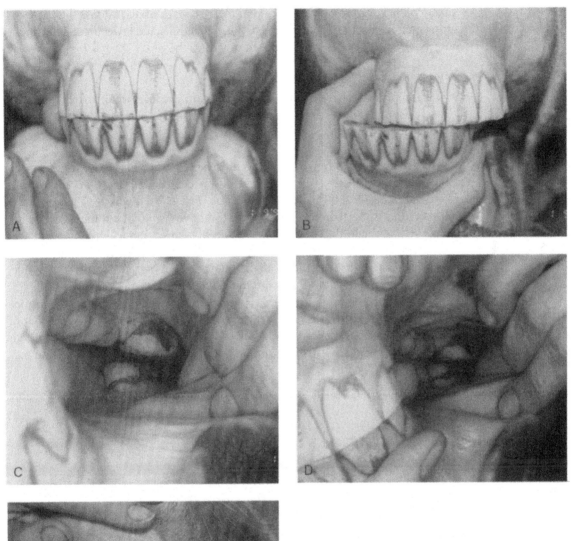

Figure 4.25 A. This horse had overlong incisors that were diagnosed by (**B**) the excessive amount of incisor contact when the mandible is moved laterally and (**C**) the gap seen between the molar arcades when the mouth is closed. **D.** After incisor bite realignment. The gap between the cheek teeth is gone. **E.** Cheek teeth come into occlusion when the mandible is moved less than 5 mm laterally.

meet. You have already determined that there is a lack of occlusion either by measuring incisor slide or by seeing a gap between the upper and lower arcades. Estimate how much incisor needs to be removed to reduce the gap.

KEY POINT

▶ It is important to have the horse's head at your eye level when visually examining incisor alignment. Looking with your head tilted down, up, or cocked to one side will distort the appearance of the incisors.

When more than 2 mm of tooth needs to be removed, conserve your energy by using power instruments. A diamond cut-off wheel mounted to a rotary motor with a flexible shaft is ideal for making a guide line (*Fig. 4.26*). If you use a wheel whose cutting radius is less than the width of the tooth, you will not cut the palate or the tongue behind the teeth. The tooth will be deeply scored and will have to be cut off with incisor nippers or ground off with a burr (*Fig. 4.27*). When using a wheel that will cut all the way through the tooth, have an assistant pull the tongue to one side, and use the thumb of your other hand to push the palate out of the way.

How you use the diamond wheel is important to both the longevity of your motor and to the heat generated while cutting. Avoid pushing the wheel faster than it can cut. This stresses the motor and will cause cementum, dentin, and enamel to build up on the wheel. Clean the diamond grit on the wheel when you see tooth ma-

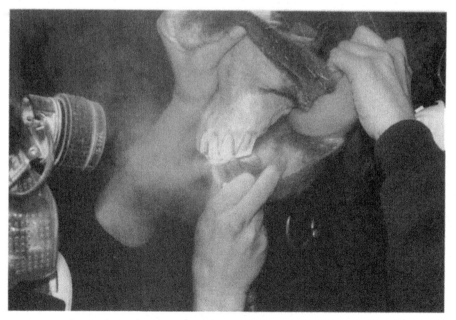

Figure 4.26 If more than 1/8 inch of tooth needs to be removed, use a diamond cut-off wheel.

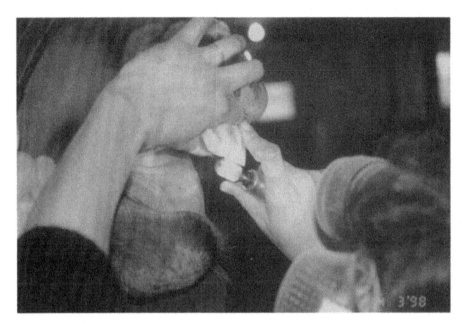

Figure 4.27 Using a cylindrical carbide burr to reduce incisors after they have been scored and nipped off. When working on upper incisors, stabilize the burr using your index finger on the premaxilla.

terial caked on it by scrubbing off the debris with water. The wheel can be water-cooled while it is in use by having an assistant drip distilled water on it or by using the clip on a water-dispensing unit made by Equi-Dent. This can make the procedure messier, but it significantly reduces friction-generated heat and airborne tooth dust.

PRACTICE TIP
Some practitioners prefer to draw the line to be cut directly on the incisors with a very-fine-tip permanent marker.

Starting your cut on a corner tooth will allow you to make a guide cut. Whether it is an upper corner incisor or lower corner incisor depends on the type of malocclusion. Remove enough to make the surface of the tooth parallel with the line of molar occlusion (*Fig. 4.28*). Next, cut the opposing tooth so that it is also parallel to this line. Repeat on the other side. Then, if you prefer to begin the main cut in the central incisors, you have an end point to cut to.

The ventral curvature (smile) is the most common incisor malocclusion (*Fig. 4.29*). Examine the incisor table angle and check molar occlusion before making any cuts. If the cheek teeth are in occlusion, then the goal is to correct the ventral curva-

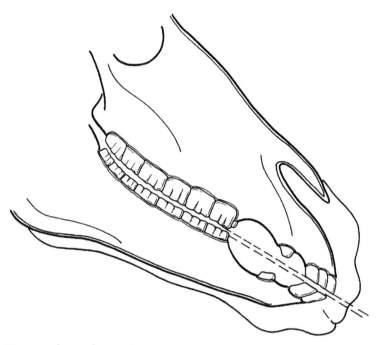

Figure 4.28 Lateral view showing how to estimate amount of incisor to be removed and how to make a guide cut parallel to the cheek teeth occlusal surface. Correction of a ventral curvature malocclusion is illustrated.

ture without significantly reducing the length of the incisors. This is done by cutting a wedge out of the dorsal central incisors (#101, #201) that reduces length in the anterior aspect of the teeth while maintaining length in the posterior aspect. The corners of #303 and #403 may also need reducing. Blend your cuts together using a burr or file after the main cuts are made.

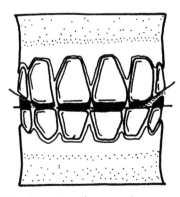

Figure 4.29 Correcting the ventral curvature malocclusion.

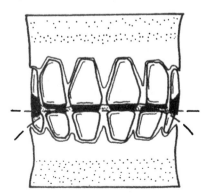

Figure 4.30 Correcting the dorsal curvature malocclusion.

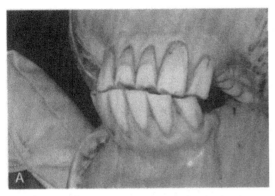 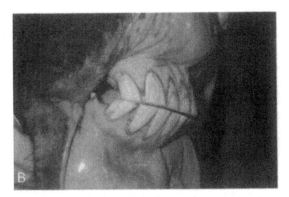

Figure 4.31 **A.** Dorsal curvature malocclusion before correction. **B.** After correction, there was a slight gap between the central incisors because #101 and #201 were so short.

The dorsal curvature (frown) malocclusion is seen when the upper central incisors are worn shorter than the lower central incisors (*4.30, 4.31A, B*). This abnormality can be created by cribbing, by trauma to the incisors, or can be associated with abnormalities in the cheek teeth. *Figure 4.30* diagrams correction of this malocclusion. When you have finished leveling the teeth, there may be a gap between the central pairs of incisors if the uppers are worn shorter than you can reduce them all to.

Slanted incisors can be seen both with and without significant cheek tooth abnormalities. Correction involves removing excess tooth at contralateral corners until the bite is horizontal. When balancing a severely slanted bite, remove a wedge-shaped piece of tooth from either corner to correct the slant, but leave the central pairs in occlusion (*Fig. 4.32*). Avoid leaving an interocclusal space between incisors.

Step malocclusion occurs secondary to incisor trauma or to missing or supernumerary teeth. There is a wide variety of types and severity (*Fig. 4.23A, B*). The goal

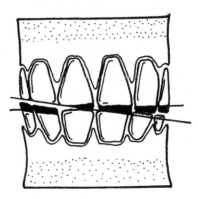

Figure 4.32 Correcting the slant malocclusion.

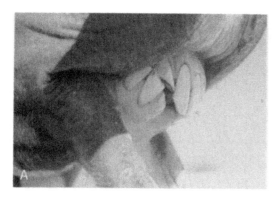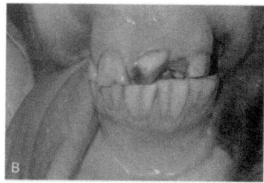

Figure 4.33   Step malocclusions of the incisors.

of correction is the same as for other types of incisor malocclusion. Determine the length the incisors need to be for them to slide laterally without getting caught on long teeth, also taking into account how much needs to be removed for proper cheek teeth occlusion.

Parrot-mouth (prognathism) and sow-mouth (brachygnathism) malocclusions allow such overgrowth of incisors that they can get caught on fences and other solid

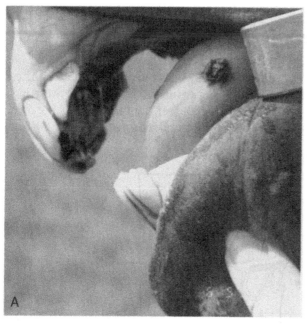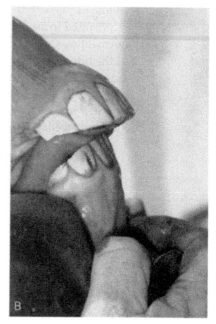

Figure 4.34   A. Parrot mouth before correction. **B.** The incisors are cut to the level of the gingiva.

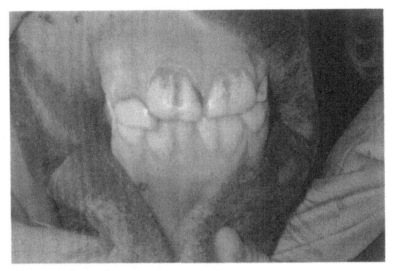

Figure 4.35 Crowded incisors in a three year old. All four of the #01 teeth have erupted. Tooth #202 is crowding #201.

objects the horse may play with. Cut the incisors as close to the gum line as possible without getting into the pulp, and keep the incisors short (*Fig. 4.34A, B*).

Overcrowding of incisors can occur when deciduous teeth are being shed and permanent teeth are erupting (*Fig. 4.35*). If the deciduous tooth is not ready to be shed, use a very thin diamond cut-off wheel to cut a vertical slice or wedge out of the tooth surfaces that are impinging on each other (*Fig. 4.36A, B*). If the permanent tooth is coming in completely behind the deciduous tooth, then the deciduous tooth must be extracted to allow the permanent tooth to move into place.

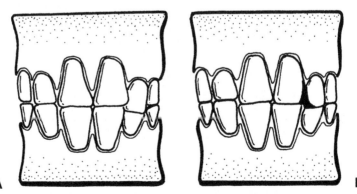

Figure 4.36 **A.** Overcrowded incisors in a 3-year-old tooth. #202 is crowding #201. **B.** After removing the contacting surfaces, tooth #201 can erupt normally. The incisors should also be leveled at this time. Cut a small amount off the corners of the teeth that are crowded to free up eruption.

After you have cut the tooth, remove the cut portions by nipping them off with incisor cutters or side nippers. Smooth the cut surface and restore the incisor angle using a 5/8-inch cylindrical burr or a drum burr, the Power Float, or an incisor rasp. Finally, some practitioners like to "dress" the labial edges of the teeth for a more professional and polished look. This procedure is similar to floating the buccal edges of the cheek teeth. Put another way, it is similar to how a farrier dresses the edge of the hoof wall.

When you are finished, the incisors should meet evenly and slide smoothly, and molar contact should be apparent with an incisor slide of approximately 5 mm in each direction. It is not unusual for horses to not have an equal amount of incisor slide on each side. For example, there may be a 3-mm slide to the right side and a 7-mm slide to the left side.

If, by accident or misjudgment, an interocclusal gap is created, the horse should be monitored for signs of discomfort due to the increased pressure on the cheek teeth and the TMJ. If the horse is reluctant to masticate, nonsteroidal anti-inflammatory medication is recommended. Abnormal mastication may predispose the horse to an impaction, so hay cubes, soaked hay pellets, or Purina Senior diet should be offered.

■ ■ SUGGESTED READING

Gaughan EM, Debowes RM. The Veterinary Clinics of North America. Dentistry. Vol. 14. Philadelphia: Saunders, 1998.
Baker GJ, Easley J. Equine Dentistry. Philadelphia: Saunders, 1999.

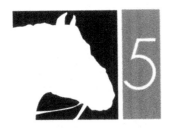

NEWBORN, WEANLING, AND ADOLESCENT HORSE DENTISTRY

PATRICIA PENCE AND KRISTIN WILEWSKI

The benefits of early dental examinations and prophylactic procedures have long been recognized in human pediatric dentistry. The goal of young horse dentistry is to detect abnormalities early so that they can be corrected or minimized before the permanent teeth are fully erupted.

Between the ages of 2 years 6 months and 5 years, horses lose 24 deciduous teeth and erupt 36 to 44 (depending on whether four canine teeth and four wolf teeth are present). At this critical time, asynchronous loss and eruption of opposing deciduous teeth can create lifelong occlusal abnormalities if not corrected. Correction of most occlusal abnormalities of cheek teeth at this stage of development is relatively simple. Teeth that are delayed in eruption can quickly (usually within weeks) erupt to be level with the arcade if the overlong opposing teeth are reduced.

Routine floating can make a profound difference in the overall health of the young horse. Young horses seem especially intolerant of oral discomfort. Seemingly minor irritation by sharp points or loose deciduous teeth can seriously impair mastication. The resulting maldigestion can manifest as poor haircoat, failure to gain weight, and episodes of colic.

■ ■ CONGENITAL DEFECTS

Congenital defects are created by either genetic or environmental factors, or occasionally a combination of both. Genetically derived defects are inheritable to varying degrees, which can create an ethical dilemma for the practitioner when making recommendations to the horse owner regarding the affected animal's fate.

A 13-year survey reported 608 foals with congenital defects; 4.3% had craniofacial malformations, and 4% had cleft palate.[1] Two equine studies reported that parrot mouth occurs at a rate of 2 to 5%.[2,3]

Occasionally, a trend traces the defect to either the sire or the dam (e.g., parrot mouth in the offspring of a thoroughbred stallion). However, most congenital defects of the head involve multiple genes, which makes predicting the chances of the defect recurring difficult, if not impossible.[4] One equine practitioner suggested this strategy: When breeding horses with no history of a certain defect in their bloodlines, and these horses produce a single offspring with a genetic defect, simply do not breed those horses with each other again.[5]

Prenatal environmental factors that can cause different genetic defects in horses include ingestion of certain toxic plants by the mare (*Astragalus mollisimus, Sorghum vulgare*),[6,7] exposure to teratogenic drugs or chemicals (cambendazole, a parasiticide),[8] fetal hormonal disorders (hypothyroidism),[9] and malpositioning of the foal in the uterus.[10] Postnatal environmental factors that can affect the head and jaws include nutrition and trauma.

Wry Nose

Wry nose is the congenital deviation of the maxilla, incisive bone, and nasal septum *(Fig. 5.1)*. This defect is thought to be inherited; however, abnormal positioning of the fetus in the uterus has also been reported to cause facial deformities.[1,11] In severe cases, suckling ability and breathing are impaired. Functional and cosmetic results can occasionally be achieved, but they require two separate surgeries several months apart.[11]

Cleft Palate

Cleft palate presents as a longitudinal defect in the hard palate, the soft palate, or both. Visualization may be difficult if the condition is limited to the soft palate. The initial clinical sign is dribbling milk after suckling. Depression, coughing, and aspiration pneumonia are also seen. Prognosis is poor with or without surgery. Without surgery, aspiration pneumonia is a serious problem. Surgical correction of this defect is difficult, and complications are common.[12]

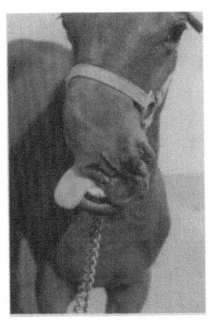

Figure 5.1 Wry nose. (Reprinted with permission from Knottenbelt DC. Colour Atlas of Diseases and Disorders of the Horse. New York: Mosby, 1994.)

Incisor Malocclusions

Congenital incisor malocclusions are relatively common in the horse. Malocclusions include forms of mandibular brachygnathism; overjet and overbite (parrot mouth); mandibular prognathism; and underbite (sow mouth, monkey mouth). Brachygnathism can occur in any breed; however, it seems to be more common in thoroughbreds and quarter horses *(Fig. 5.2)*. Prognathism can also be seen in any breed, but it is more common in ponies and miniature horses *(Fig. 5.3)*. Prognathism in miniature horses may be genetically associated with the achondroplastic dwarfism condition.[13–15]

These malocclusions can be attributed to abnormalities in the maxilla, the mandible, or both.[16] Abnormalities may be limited to malocclusion of the incisors, or they may occur in combination with varying degrees of malocclusion of the upper and lower cheek teeth arcades.[5]

KEY POINT:
▶ Early recognition and treatment of incisor malocclusions is necessary for successful correction. The foal needs to be at least 10 weeks old but less than 6 months old to attain the maximum amount of correction.[17,18]

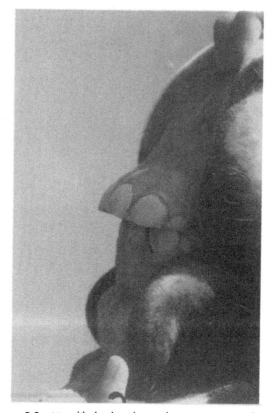

Figure 5.2 Mandibular brachygnathism in a quarter horse.

KEY POINT:
▶ With the exception of brachygnathism (parrot mouth) and prognathism (sow mouth, monkey mouth), most congenital defects of the dentition are subtle and go undetected until the foal is older.

Supernumerary, Malerupted, and Missing Teeth

Supernumerary teeth are teeth in excess of the normal expected number.[19] Although they are usually not recognized until the horse is several months or years old, supernumerary teeth are considered a congenital condition because they result from inappropriate differentiation of dental germinal tissue during gestational development.[20] It is more common for excess incisors to appear than excess molars. Supernumerary incisors rarely cause problems. If they do not wear normally, they can be cut or floated.

The most common presentation of a supernumerary cheek tooth is as a fourth molar. This tooth may erupt lingually or buccally to the other teeth if there is no room for it in the arcade.[20] Because they are not opposed by a tooth in the opposite arcade, these teeth require at least annual reduction to prevent soft-tissue injury.

Maleruptions can occur with any tooth, but the third cheek tooth is most commonly implicated.[21,23] The third cheek tooth (#8) of each arcade is the last permanent tooth to erupt and must enter between the firmly imbedded second and fourth cheek teeth. Lack of sufficient space between those two teeth may cause the third cheek tooth to erupt lingually or laterally, or may prevent eruption altogether. When eruption is totally impaired, a progressive swelling appears over the apex of the tooth, and this tooth may develop secondary apical osteitis, infection, and fistula formation. This condition can occur in mandibular or maxillary teeth.

Occasionally, teeth may develop normally but in an abnormal position. Horizontally impacted teeth have been reported.[24] As these teeth grow and roots develop, they can cause deformation of the face and disturb growth of adjacent teeth *(Fig. 5.4)*.

Missing teeth of a congenital nature are caused by lack of formation or maldevelopment of the tooth bud *(Fig. 5.5)*. The tooth may be absent, or a mass of dental

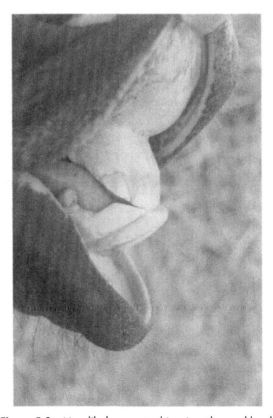

Figure 5.3 Mandibular prognathism in a thoroughbred.

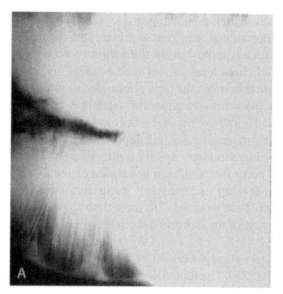
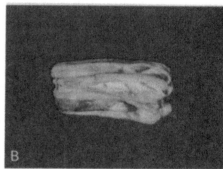

Figure 5.4 **A.** Horizontally impacted tooth #206. **B.** This is the horizontally impacted tooth in **A.** removed by lateral buccotomy.

tissue with no defined structure may be present within the jaw. This amorphous mass grows but cannot erupt; therefore, no tooth is present in the arcade.[24] It appears as a lump within the jaw that may or may not be accompanied by a fistula. After birth, the condition is usually secondary to trauma. Missing teeth are a problem because the other teeth in the arcade shift to fill in the empty space, which in turn creates small spaces between them that allow food to accumulate. The teeth in the opposing arcade are also affected. Any unopposed occlusal surfaces will erupt into the empty spaces.

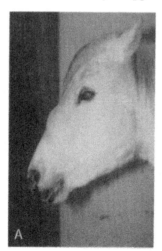
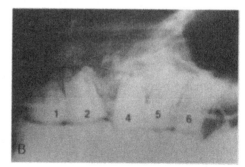

Figure 5.5 A. Facial swelling caused by maleruption of unformed dental tissue dorsal to arcade appeared at 5 years of age. B. Radiographic appearance of dental tissue in A. Effect on the arcade was similar to that of a missing tooth. (Reprinted with permission from Knottenbelt DC. Colour Atlas of Diseases and Disorders of the Horse. New York: Mosby, 1994.)

Congenital Tumors and Cysts

Although rare, congenital tumors and bone cysts can appear in weanling and adolescent horses. Oral and dental neoplasia are more common in young horses than in older ones.[22] Any firm, noninflamed swelling should be investigated to rule out bone cysts and neoplasia. Diagnosis is made through clinical appearance, radiography, and biopsy. Primary dental tumors are classified by the type of tissues they contain. Ameloblastic odontomas have been seen in the maxillae of foals *(Fig. 5.6)*.[25,26]

Osseous, cystlike swellings in the maxillae and mandibles of young horses have been documented.[27,28] Because of their nature to grow and expand, these structures can be destructive. Teeth may be displaced or their development impaired, the maxillary sinuses may be invaded, and the structural integrity of the maxilla or mandible may be threatened. Juvenile ossifying fibromas are tumor like masses that develop in the rostral mandible of horses 2 months to 2 years old *(Fig. 5.7)*.[29] Although not malignant, these masses are locally invasive and expansive. Surgical excision and radiation therapy have been used successfully to treat some cases.[30]

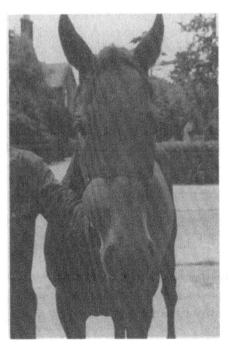

Figure 5.6 Facial swelling caused by an ameloblastoma. (Reprinted with permission from Baker GJ, Easley J, eds. Equine Dentistry. Philadelphia: WB Saunders, 1999.)

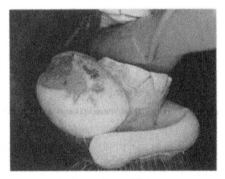

Figure 5.7 Juvenile ossifying fibroma in a 14-month-old thoroughbred. The superficial ulceration only developed late in the condition. (Reprinted with permission from Baker GJ, Easley J, eds. Equine Dentistry. Philadelphia: WB Saunders, 1999.)

Dentigerous cysts (e.g., temporal odontoma, heterotropic polydontia, ear tooth) are benign congenital tumors that appear in the temporal region of the head.[31] They are composed of varying amounts of dental tissues within a cystic structure that has a secretory epithelial lining. The secretory tissue produces a mucoid discharge that drains from a fistulous tract. Contrast radiography helps determine the full extent of the structure. Although these cysts are usually minimally disfiguring, surgical excision is recommended because serious infections of the cyst have developed in some cases.[22]

■ ■   NEWBORN TO 1 YEAR OLD

Routine Dental Care

Horses in this age group should have an oral examination performed during the neonatal period and about every 3 months thereafter. They should be examined for congenital defects, proper growth of the maxilla and mandible, alignment of the upper and lower arcades, supernumerary teeth, and congenital tumors and cysts. Frequent examinations are necessary because occasionally foals are born with normal incisor occlusion but develop malocclusions during periods of rapid growth. Some congenital defects and growth abnormalities can be corrected if treated before the foal is 6 months old. However, because congenital defects of the head and jaws are widely considered to be heritable, the ethics of correcting these conditions in breeding animals can be an issue.[4,32,33]

Routine dental care (i.e., floating) can be started at 4–6 months of age and should be scheduled every 3–4 months. Hooks or ramps on the #6s may be present at this time and can easily be filed level. Do not over float these soft teeth. A full-mouth speculum can be used, but be careful to not open the mouth too wide. Tranquilization makes the dental less traumatic for the foal.

PRACTICE TIP:

Miniature horse floats are ideal for young horses with small heads.

KEY POINT:

▶ Deciduous teeth are somewhat softer than permanent teeth. Sharp points form faster on the buccal edges of deciduous maxillary teeth and the lingual edges of mandibular teeth than they do in permanent teeth.

Parrot Mouth

In addition to congenital brachygnathia, acquired brachygnathia has been reported in foals between 1 and 6 months of age.[5,17] These foals were born with normal incisor occlusion but have overbites on later examinations *(Fig. 5.8)*. Uneven devel-

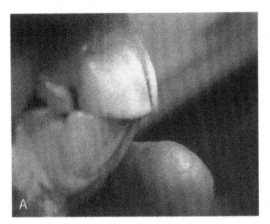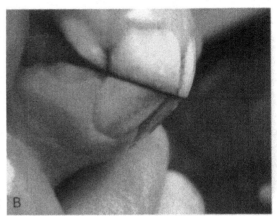

Figure 5.8 **A.** The abnormally rostral angle of eruption in this corner incisor was promoting an acquired overbite condition. **B.** The overbite self-corrected when the corner incisors were reduced and the other incisors balanced. (Photos courtesy of Tony Basile.)

opment of the maxilla and mandible during periods of rapid growth, trauma to the temporomandibular area, and mating animals with radically dissimilar head types are possible causes. The possibility of these changes occurring in foals that were normal at birth underscores the necessity for frequent examinations during the first year.

Regardless of whether the brachygnathic condition is congenital or acquired, parrot mouth can be improved, even corrected in some cases. Correction of parrot mouth requires inhibiting the rostral growth of the maxilla and premaxilla, preventing the incisors and incisive bones from curling down over the mandible, and encouraging the rostral growth of the mandible. See *Box 5.1* for the principles of orthodontic management of parrot mouth. The application of temporary wire tension bands to the first maxillary cheek teeth are used to retard growth of the maxilla and premaxilla *(Fig. 5.9A and B)*.[17,18,34] Rostral growth of the mandible is encouraged by two things: an orthodontic appliance is used to put a flat barrier between the upper and lower incisors, so the uppers cannot entrap the lowers. The cheek teeth are

---

BOX 5.1   PRINCIPLES OF ORTHODONTIC MANAGEMENT OF PARROT MOUTH[5]
1. Prevent or reduce abnormal wear of the teeth.
2. Prevent or correct downward gravitational drift of the incisive bone and upper incisor teeth.
3. Inhibit rostral growth of the maxilla and premaxilla.
4. Encourage rostral growth of the mandible.

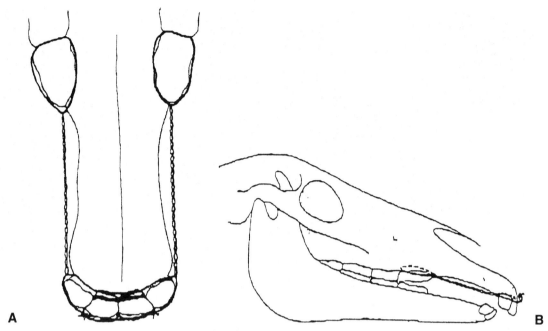

Figure 5.9 **A.** Ventrodorsal view of the temporary premaxillary tension band device. **B.** Lateral view of the temporary premaxillary tension band device. (Reprinted with permission from Gift LJ, De Bowes RM, Clem MF, et al. Brachygnathia in horses: 20 cases [1979–1989]. J Am Vet Med Assoc 1992;200:715.)

floated, and any conformational abnormality that would prevent normal mastication and free motion of the mandible is corrected.[5]

The simplest appliance is the bite plate *(Fig. 5.10)*. It consists of a flat piece of plastic or metal that is held between the incisors to prevent the upper incisors from inhibiting rostral motion and growth of the mandible. It is attached to the halter and removed for short periods to allow the foal to eat. More sophisticated fixed devices have also been used.[5]

Lack of incisor wear makes frequent incisor trims necessary. The incisors need to be short enough to allow free lateral movement of the jaw. Hooks, ramps, and excessive transverse ridges need to be reduced as well because they can inhibit rostral movement of the mandible.

Conservative therapy for parrot mouth in foals involves application of a bite plate and frequent dentals to prevent any inhibition of rostral growth of the mandible.

Young, rapidly growing foals on a high-energy diet that develop brachyngnathia during a rapid growth period should be placed on a balanced ration with total digestible energy adjusted to meet National Research Council (NRC) requirements for growth.[20]

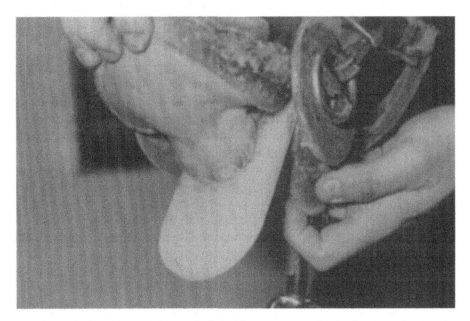

Figure 5.10 A bite plate may be applied to reduce or prevent the development of an overbite lesion and allow for possible correction of an overjet lesion. (Reprinted with permission from DeBowes RM, Gaughan EM. Congenital Dental Disease in Horses. Vet Clin North Am Equine Pract 1998;14:279.)

YEARLINGS TO 2 YEAR OLDS

Routine Dental Care

When the yearling reaches 12 months of age, all the deciduous teeth should have erupted and the first permanent cheek teeth (the #9s) are starting to erupt. Sharp points will have formed on the deciduous cheek teeth (#6–8). Hooks or ramps may have formed on the #6s and need to be corrected. Dental examinations should be scheduled every 3–4 months, and teeth should be floated as needed.

For many yearlings, floating is all that is necessary. Because the teeth are soft, you may prefer to use carbide chip blades instead of solid carbide blades. If solid carbide blades are used, very little pressure should be applied, and the teeth should be inspected frequently to prevent overfloating. If there are sharp points on the #9s, they can be smoothed with an S file.

The occlusal surfaces are very corrugated in young horses and should not be mistaken for excessive transverse ridges. Do not overfloat the arcades and remove all the corrugation. Bit seats can be created if the horse will be bitted before the next dental visit.

Wolf teeth should be extracted at this age if they can be palpated. The wolf teeth go through the gumline at 6 months of age in most horses. If no wolf teeth are visible, palpate the gum rostral to the #6s to feel for unerupted or impacted wolf teeth. Occasionally, these teeth erupt in abnormal positions and can be found lying sideways under the gingiva. Lower wolf teeth are rare, but each horse should be checked for them. Lower wolf teeth can cause severe bitting problems. Techniques to extract wolf teeth are discussed in Chapter 4, Basic Dental Techniques.

All deciduous incisors should be present by 12 months of age. At this age, the incisors may not need any work, but they should be examined for proper eruption and alignment. If imbalances are found, the overlong incisors can be reduced by burring or filing as described for minor incisor bite realignment.

Horses that avulse an incisor without completely removing it can have it wired back into place if the problem is recognized early enough. Ideally, the tooth should be wired within 6 hours of the trauma. If extensive bone damage occurs or if the tissue is necrotic, extraction is the only choice. When in doubt, try to save the tooth—it can always be extracted later. Refer to the chapter on dental infections for more information on treatment.

If the tooth bud is damaged, the permanent tooth may fail to develop, or a deformed permanent tooth may erupt at a different rate from the rest of the incisors. Both situations create a malalignment that needs to be corrected on a regular basis.

KEY POINT:
▶ **Trauma to the young horse's deciduous teeth or jaw can affect the development of the permanent teeth.**

2 TO 4 YEAR OLDS

The dentition of the horse is in its most dynamic state when the horse is between 2 and 5 years of age. Horses in this age group are continuously shedding deciduous teeth as the permanent teeth erupt. Horses shed 24 teeth and erupt 36 to 44 teeth by the time they are 5 years old *(Table 5.1)*.

Asymetric Eruption

If opposing deciduous caps are not shed at approximately the same time, the occlusal surfaces of the arcades can become so uneven that mastication is difficult *(Fig. 5.11)*. For example, if a horse loses the #208 tooth at 3 years 8 months of age, the permanent tooth will erupt and be level with the arcade 2 months later. If, however, the #308 is not shed until 3 years 10 months of age, the permanent #208 will be at the gum line when the permanent #208 is level with the arcade. One month later, the #208 will be longer than the rest of the arcade, and the #308 will be shorter. The overlong #208 will prevent normal lateral excursion and interfere with mastication. In addition, this overlong tooth makes it difficult for the horse

TABLE 5.1   **Eruption Schedule**

Teeth (in order of eruption)	Eruption Age
Deciduous	
#1 First incisor	Birth–first week
#2 Second incisor	4–6 weeks
#3 Third incisor	6–9 months
#6 Second premolar	Birth–first 2 weeks
#7 Third premolar	Birth–first 2 weeks
#8 Fourth premolar	Birth–first 2 weeks
Permanent	
#4 First premolar (wolf tooth)	6–9 months
#9 First molar	9–15 months
#1 First incisor	2.5 years
#6 Second premolar	2 years 8 months
#7 Third premolar	2 years 10 months
#10 Second molar	2–3 years
#2 Second incisor	3.5 years
#11 Third molar	3.5–4 years
#8 Fourth premolar	3 years 8 months
#3 Third incisor	4.5 years

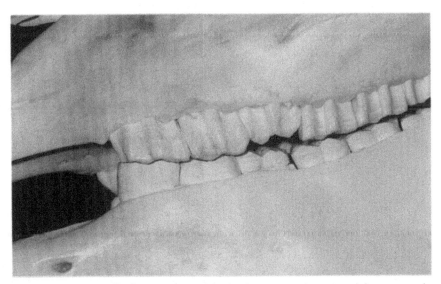

Figure 5.11   An example of asymmetric eruption. The #108 and #208 teeth have erupted and will be level with the arcade soon, but the #308 and #408 have retained deciduous teeth. In the live horse, the #308 and #408 permanent teeth would still be just barely breaking through the gums. The retained deciduous teeth put tremendous pressure on the permanent teeth in the opposing arcade as well as the permanent teeth on which they lie.

to bend at the poll as it locks into space left by the short tooth. These imbalances can be prevented by regular dental care timed with the eruption schedule of the permanent dentition.

Gingivitis and Trauma

Tooth eruption can be accompanied by varying degrees of gingivitis and trauma. The sharp edges of the cap roots irritate the gingiva during mastication. Lingual points on unworn, permanent mandibular cheek teeth can become long and sharp enough to cause trauma to the tongue and gingiva of the palate if they are not floated *(Fig. 5.12)*. The buccal mucosa opposite the #11s can be injured by sharp points in 3 year olds.

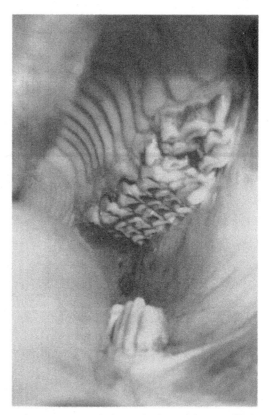

Figure 5.12   The long, sharp points on the lingual edges of the mandibular teeth were irritating the gingiva at the palatal aspects of teeth #107 and 207. The deciduous tooth had not been shed yet, which added to the irritation. Treatment for this case of gingivitis involved removing retained deciduous teeth and floating the sharp points.

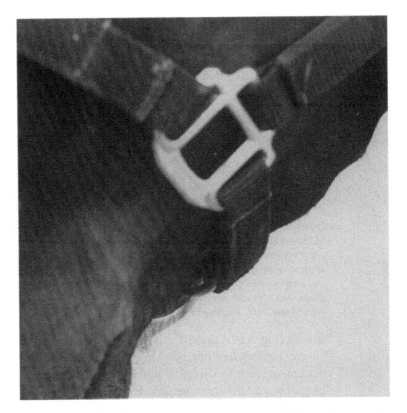

Figure 5.13 Eruption bumps or pseudo cysts on ventral mandible of a 3½-year-old mare.

Periostitis

Periostitis, inflammation of the periosteum, can occur when retained deciduous premolars impede the eruption of the permanent teeth. As the permanent teeth mature, the reserve crown grows in the apical direction. Pressure exerted on the cortical bone of the mandible or maxilla by the expanding tooth causes lysis of the bone overlying the apex. The cortical bone itself may expand to produce bumps under the mandible or over the bridge of the nose; these bumps are called eruption cysts or pseudocysts *(Fig. 5.13)* In most cases, these swellings spontaneously resolve when the overlying deciduous tooth is shed, allowing the permanent tooth to erupt.

Impacted Teeth

The #8s are the most common teeth to become impacted because they are the last teeth to erupt. One author believed that impaction of the #308 and 408 is the most important cause of apical osteitis and subsequent formation of mandibular dental

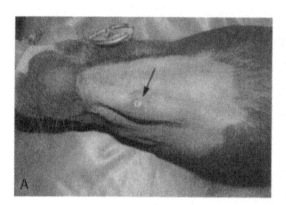
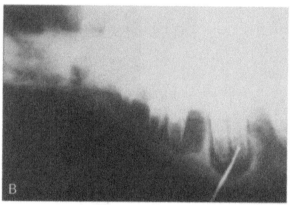

Figure 5.14 **A.** Firm, nonpainful swelling and draining sinus tract in the mandible over the root of tooth #307. The draining sinus had been present for several years, and the swelling became progressively larger. **B.** Oblique radiograph of the mandibile of a horse suffering from a chronic swelling and discharging sinus tract over the root of the third lower cheek tooth. A probe has been inserted into the tract. This is the typical appearance of chronic apical abscessation. (Reprinted with permission from Knottenbelt DC. Colour Atlas of Diseases and Disorders of the Horse New York: Mosby, 1994.)

fistulae *(Fig. 5.14 A and B)*.[23] If the space between the #7 and #9 is inadequate, the #8 may be displaced lingually (lower arcade) or palatally (upper arcade). This displacement creates an irregular lingual or palatal arcade surface, which allows food to be packed into the area where the tooth should have erupted, eventually resulting in periodontal disease.

Some authors have suggested that one of the more common causes of impacted permanent cheek teeth are the presence of rostral hooks and ramps on the #6s.[2,5] Rostral hooks on the #6 deciduous teeth apply caudally directed pressure to the opposing #6 teeth, which is transmitted to the #7s and #8s *(Fig. 5.15a and b)*. This abnormally directed pressure can wedge the deciduous teeth in place, preventing them from shedding normally.

The retained deciduous teeth cause great hydrostatic pressure to build up in the expanding apical region of the permanent teeth. The apical region becomes inflamed and susceptible to trauma and hematogenous colonization of bacteria.[35,36]

Treating impacted teeth involves grinding down the mesial and distal contact points on the impacted tooth and its neighbor. Preventative care involves removing rostral hooks and ramps, removing caps in a timely manner, balancing the erupted teeth, and floating off sharp points so that lateral excursion is more comfortable.

Deciduous Tooth Caps

Identifying deciduous teeth that are ready to be exfoliated is an important part of the dental care of adolescent horses. As mentioned previously, knowledge of the eruption schedule is required to know whether a deciduous tooth is due to be shed. For practitioners unfamiliar with working on horses of this age group, distinguishing between a deciduous tooth and a permanent tooth can be confusing. Below is a list of distinguishing characteristics between deciduous and permanent teeth.

■ ■ DISTINGUISHING DECIDUOUS TEETH FROM PERMANENT TEETH

1. Deciduous teeth are whiter than permanent teeth due to the cementum's yellowish color on the erupting permanent teeth.
2. Deciduous teeth are somewhat smaller than permanent teeth and have a distinct neck between the crown and the root. This is especially noticeable in the incisors. If the size difference is not apparent, use other distinguishing features.
3. The incisal or occlusal surfaces of deciduous teeth are normally worn flat. Permanent incisors have uneven incisal surfaces. The deep, cementum-covered enamel folds on the occlusal surface of the permanent cheek teeth contrast with the smooth, sometimes slightly wavy surface of the deciduous cheek teeth.
4. If the deciduous teeth have not been floated recently, the enamel points on the buccal surfaces of the maxillary deciduous cheek teeth and the lingual edges of the mandibular deciduous cheek teeth are very sharp compared with newly erupted permanent cheek teeth.

The following are instances when manual extraction of a deciduous cap is necessary.

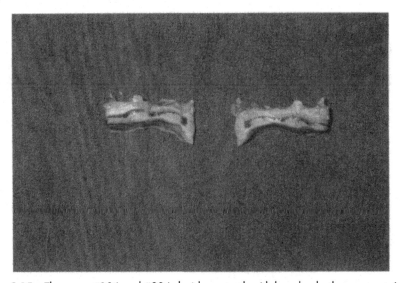

Figure 5.15 These are #106 and #206 deciduous teeth with long hooks that were retained in a colt. They were removed with the #107 and #207. The #307 and #407 deciduous teeth were also present and were difficult to extract due to prolonged caudal pressure on the #306 and #406 caused by the hooks. This horse was also developing a mild overbite, which self-corrected when the caps were removed and the teeth were floated.

1. The cap has broken away from the gingival margin, i.e., a break can either be seen or felt when an instrument is rubbed along the gingival margin *(Fig. 5.16)*.
2. The cap is loose.
3. According to the eruption schedule, the cap is either ready or past due to exfoliate on its own.

KEY POINT

▶ If the cap is firmly attached and has no break at the gingival margin, recheck it in 2 weeks. Exposing a permanent tooth before it has sufficiently matured can seriously damage the maturation of the infundibular cementum.[32] If no changes have occurred within 4 weeks, then a radiographic examination should be performed to determine whether a permanent tooth is present.

Two different situations can present themselves when deciduous incisor caps are being extracted. The first, more common situation is when the permanent tooth

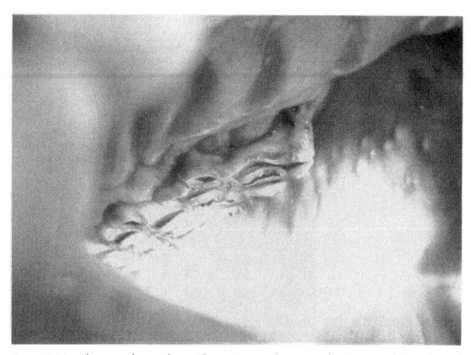

Figure 5.16 Close-up photo taken with an intra-oral camera showing an obvious line of demarcation between the deciduous tooth and the permanent tooth. (Photo courtesy of Tony Basile.)

lies directly beneath the cap, allowing normal deciduous root absorption to occur. In the second situation, the deciduous incisor is overdue to be shed or the permanent tooth is crowded or impacted. In this case, the permanent tooth erupts caudally to the deciduous tooth. Normal deciduous root absorption cannot occur under these circumstances. The root may be partially absorbed or completely intact (Case Report #1).

To remove an incisor cap that has a break at the gingival margin, grasp the cap firmly with incisor forceps. Pull down with a slightly outward twisting motion for the upper incisors and up with the same twisting motion for the lowers. Extract any root fragments left in the gingiva with root fragment forceps. Loose flaps of gingiva can be excised with either a scalpel or scissors.

Extracting deciduous incisors that have permanent teeth erupting caudally is a more surgical procedure. Sedation should be given if the horse was not sedated already. A 2% lidocaine local anesthestic is injected into the gingiva overlying the deciduous root, which usually appears as a slightly raised and blanched area. Make an incision over the root with a #15 scalpel blade, and with a root elevator break down any soft tissue or periosteal attachments that hold the deciduous root in place. The tooth can be extracted whole if the root has been completely elevated. Rinse the cavity with dilute antiseptic, and give a tetanus booster if necessary. Examine the incisors adjacent to the caudally displaced tooth to make sure that there is room for the tooth to move forward.

Overcrowding can occur in incisors when there is insufficient room for the permanent tooth or teeth to erupt. It is more common in ponies and miniatures (see Chapter 8 Miniature Horse Dentistry). For example, when the permanent #1s erupt, they should be checked for overcrowding by the deciduous #2s. If the #2s appear to be crowding the #1s, they can be clipped on their medial sides to create more room for the permanent #1s. This can be done with either a side-cutter or a Dremel instrument fitted with a cut-off wheel. A small section of tooth is sliced off in a vertical plane and removed with forceps (Case Report #2).

KEY POINT:
▶ Overcrowding occurs when there is not enough room for the permanent teeth to erupt. This can be caused by retained deciduous teeth, small jaw size, trauma, or the presence of supernumerary teeth.

Most cheek teeth caps can be removed with a set of upper or lower Reynolds cap extractors. However, some situations may be easier if specialty instruments are used. More refined dental instruments have been designed by World Wide Equine specifically for extracting upper deciduous cheek teeth and for extracting lower deciduous cheek teeth.

The #6 caps are extracted using upper or lower premolar cap forceps depending on the tooth's location. Grasp the cap firmly with the forceps, rock it slightly side to side, and remove it by rocking it off the buccal edge and pulling lingually and down (see Fig 5.1).

KEY POINT:
▶ It is more difficult to remove root slivers from the buccal gingival margin, so specific efforts are made to create an especially clean break on that side. Rock deciduous cheek teeth off the buccal attachment and into the mouth.

The #7 deciduous caps are extracted the same way if they are really loose. Because the #7s are wedged between the #6s and #8s, they may be a little harder to remove. A long, flat-head screw driver can be introduced into the break at the gingival margin and then twisted to pop that edge of the cap down. Alternatively, the tip of the screwdriver can be inserted between the #6 and #7, using the #6 as a leverage point (see Fig 5.2). Finally, any overlong cheek teeth that are not caps ready for extraction should be reduced.

PRACTICE TIP:
A long, flat-head screwdriver can be used to loosen #7 or #8 deciduous cheek teeth that are wedged firmly in place.

KEY POINT:
▶ If the attachment of the deciduous tooth root at the gingival margin is disrupted, the cap is ready to be removed.

If deciduous teeth are not being shed in the correct sequence, the caps should be pulled off the late-erupting teeth if the permanent tooth has erupted through the gum. For example, if the horse recently lost the #106 cap and the remaining #6 caps are ready to extract, it should have already shed the deciduous #1s. If the #1s are still present, they are late and should be extracted along with the loose #6s. The permanent #1s will be visible at the gumline (see Case Report #1).

■ ■   **2 YEAR OLDS**

Routine Dentistry
The #1s (central incisors) should be shed at 2 years 6 months of age. Two months later, at 2 years 8 months, the #6s should be shed. Two months after the #6s are shed, at 2 years 10 months, the #7s should be ready to come off. Dental examinations should ideally be scheduled every 2 months, from age 2 years 6 months to 3 years. These examinations should ensure that these teeth are shed at the right time, these enabling equal eruption of permanent teeth. The second molars (#10s) erupt at variable times during the period between 2 and 3 years of age.

■■   3 YEAR OLDS

Routine Dentistry

Dental requirements of 3 year olds are similar to those of the horse between 2 years 6 months and 3 years. The difference is that one fewer set of teeth are shed. Retained deciduous caps, overlong teeth, malalignment, and overcrowding can be seen at this age.

The #2s (middle incisors) should be shed at 3 years 6 months of age. Two months later, at 3 years 8 months of age, the #8s should be ready to come off. Dental examinations should be scheduled accordingly to be sure that these teeth are shed at the appropriate times, allowing normal and equal eruption of permanent teeth. Unlike the central incisors, the middle incisors in some horses may not be ready to come off until after the #8s are shed. The third molars (#11s) should erupt sometime in the latter half of the third year.

KEY POINT:
▶ Some 3 year olds will shed the #8 teeth before they shed the #2 teeth.

Any overlong cheek teeth are reduced as described in Chapter 4, Basic Dental Techniques. The most common overlong cheek teeth in 3 year olds are the #109s, #209s, #306s, and #406s. Some horses may also have hooks on #106 and #206 if the mandible and maxilla are slightly anisognathic. Reduce overlong teeth, restore table angles, float sharp points, put in bit seats, and reduce and align incisors as necessary.

While most 3 year olds only need minor, if any, incisor reduction, be sure to check molar occlusion after all cheek tooth work has been done. The occasional horse will need a major bite realignment in which the incisors must be cut and burred or filed to achieve adequate molar occlusion (see Case Reports #2 and #3).

■■   4 YEAR OLDS

Routine Dentistry

Four year olds have only one set of deciduous teeth to lose, the #3s (corner incisors). The #3s should be ready to shed at 4 years 6 months of age. The #11s are also erupting at this time, and they may cause some discomfort as they cut through the gingiva.

Dental examinations and appropriate work should be scheduled every 4 to 6 months. The jaws are still growing in length and depth, and the #3s and #11s are erupting. Complete dentals in this age group are the same as for any age. Overlong cheek teeth need to be reduced and have table angles restored, sharp points on all teeth should be floated, bit seats should be put in if desired, and incisors should be reduced if necessary. The most common overlong teeth in this age group are the

#109, 110, 209, 210, 306, 406, and sometimes the #308 and 408. Hooks on the #106 and 206 may also be seen.

Overlong or uneven incisors are most often caused by unequal eruption secondary to delayed or unequal shedding of deciduous teeth. Uneven incisors can be leveled by the use of an incisor rasp or a cylindrical burr on a Dremel motor or similar unit. Take care to prevent damage to the palate, which is close to the incisal surface at this age. Reduce the overlong incisors until they are level with the adjacent teeth. If the incisors are level and there is too much contact after the cheek teeth have been corrected; in this case, a minor (or major, if necessary) incisor reduction must be performed on all the incisors.

Some horses at this age cannot be brought into full molar contact, and some incisor contact remains after the full dental, including incisor bite realignment. These horses should be checked in 30 to 60 days for molar contact because the rapid eruption of permanent cheek teeth often brings these teeth back into occlusion. If too much incisor contact is still present, more reduction of the incisors can be done at this time.

Case Report #1

This is a 2-year, 8-month-old American Saddlebred mare in show training. In the photos taken on the day of the initial dental visit (see color plates 28 through 30), it is apparent that this mare has #106 and #206 cap fragments that were ready for extraction. Palpation showed that the #306 and #406 caps were loosening and were also ready for extraction. Sharp points were also present on all arcades. Examination of the central incisors, the #1s, however, revealed that the deciduous teeth had not been shed and the permanent teeth were late in erupting. Close inspection of the gingiva ventral to the #301 and #401 showed blanched areas where the permanent teeth were erupting. That day, the #1 and #6 caps were removed, sharp points on all arcades were floated, and the incisors were filed until good occlusion was achieved.

Debris obscured visibility of the permanent #1s and #6s the day after the initial dental, but the permanent teeth were readily palpable.

Photographs taken 5 weeks after the initial dental show how quickly the permanent teeth erupt once the deciduous teeth are out of the way (see color plates 31 through 34). The #7 caps were extracted 1 month later, when the mare was 2 years 10 months of age, and bit seats were created on the #6s at that time.

Case Report #2

This is a Hackney pony gelding in show training. He showed dental problems encountered due to overcrowding. Overcrowded incisors are common in small muzzled horses like ponies and miniatures. In this case, the overcrowding was most evident in the lower incisors and became a problem as the permanent teeth erupted. At 3 years 6 months of age, he had a retained #302 cap contributing to overcrowding the permanent #302, which caused it to erupt in a position caudal to the arcade. The deciduous tooth was removed, and the lateral side of the permanent #301 was cut to allow more room for the permanent #302 to shift forward, which it did (see color plates 35 through 38). The #402 was also trapped behind the #401, but took longer to realign because the overcrowding was more severe in that arcade.

This horse did not have a dental scheduled as desired over the next year and was not seen again until he was 4 years 9 months of age. At that time, a retained #403 cap was contributing to overcrowding on this side of his mouth (see color plates 39 through 42). The cap was extracted at that visit. By the time the pony was 5 years 2 months of age, the incisors had shifted into as normal an alignment as his small jaws would allow (see color plates 43 through 46).

This case illustrates that removing caps in a timely manner helps prevent alignment problems in the permanent dentition. If doubt exists concerning whether a normal permanent tooth is present to replace the nonexfoliated deciduous tooth, radiographs should be taken.

Case Report #3

This case involves a 3-year, 6-month-old Paint stallion that was not responding well to training and was showing great resistance to pressure on the bit (see color plates 47 through 50). He also dribbling grain while eating. Initial examination revealed poor occlusion of the cheek teeth, sharp upper and lower enamel points, and a retained #208 cap. The remaining #8 caps had already been shed, and the #108 and opposing #408 were already in occlusion. This horse also had accentuated transverse ridges on the #109, 209, 306, 307, 406, and 407 teeth. The excess areas of the ridges were reduced, the table angle was restored, the #208 cap was removed, all arcades were floated, and bit seats were created. Occlusion was rechecked and found to be inadequate—not surprising because it was not good to begin with; a small amount of occlusal surface had been removed. With the incisors closed and held at the neutral position, the cheek teeth had a quarter-inch interocclusal gap. A full incisor bite realignment was performed, and the incisors were reduced by a quarter inch. After the incisor bite realignment, excellent occlusion was achieved. This horse's attitude improved greatly, and he no longer dribbled grain after his dental.

KEY POINT:
▶ Although young horses normally do not need major incisor reduction, all major horses should be checked for proper occlusion once the caps have been removed and the cheek teeth have been leveled and floated.

■ ■ REFERENCES

1. Crowe MW, Swerczek TW. Equine congenital defects. Am J Vet Res 1985;46:353–358.
2. Uhlinger C. Survey of selected dental abnormalities in 233 horses. In: Proceedings of the 33rd Annual Convention of the American Association of Equine Practitioners. New Orleans, LA; 1987:577–583.
3. Duke A. Equine bit analysis. Handout notes from the Annual Conference of American Veterinary Dental Society, New Orleans, 1989.
4. Emily P. The genetics of occlusion. Vet Forum 1990;6:22–23.
5. Easley J. Basic equine orthodontics. In: Baker GJ, Easley J, eds. Equine Dentistry. Philadelphia: WB Saunders, 1999.
6. McIlwraith CW, James LF. Limb deformities in foals associated with the ingestion of locoweed by mares. J Am Vet Med Assoc 1982;181:255–258.
7. Prichard JT, Voss JL. Fetal ankylosis in horses associated with hybrid Sudan pasture. J Am Vet Med Assoc 1967;150:871–873.
8. Drudge JH, Lyons E, Swerczek ET, Tolliver SC. Cambendazole for strongyle control in a pony band: selection of a drug-resistant population of small strongyles and teratologic implications. Am J Vet Res 1983;44:110–114.
9. McLaughlin BG, Doige CE, McLaughlin PS. Thyroid hormone levels in foals with congenital musculoskeletal lesions. Can Vet J 1986;27:264–267.
10. Vandeplassche M, Simoens P, Bouters R, et al. Aetiology and pathogenesis of congenital torticollis and head scoliosis in the equine fetus. Equine Vet J 1984;16:419–424.
11. Stashak TS. Wound management and reconstructive surgery of the head region. In: Stashak TS, ed. Equine Wound Management. Philadelphia: Lea & Febiger, 1991.
12. Bowman KF, Tate LP, Robertson JT. Cleft palate. In: White NA, Moore JN, eds. Current practice of equine surgery. Philadelphia: JB Lippincott, 1990.
13. Jayo M, Leipold HW, Dennis SM, Eldridge FE. Brachygnathia superior and degenerative joint disease, a new lethal syndrome in Angus calves. Vet Pathol 1987;24:148–155.
14. Lear TL, Cox JH, Kennedy GA. Autosomal trisomy in a thoroughbred colt: 65,XY, 31. Equine Vet J 1997;31:85–88.
15. McLaughlin GB, Doige LE. Congenital musculoskeletal lesions and hyperplastic goiter in foals. Can Vet J 1981;22:130.
16. Miles AEW, Grigson CL. Colyer's variations and diseases of the teeth in animals. Revised Ed. Cambridge: Cambridge University Press, 1990.
17. Gift LJ, DeBowes RM, Clem MF, et al. Brachygnathia in horses: 20 cases (1979–1989). J Am Vet Med Assoc 1992;200:715.
18. DeBowes RM. Brachygnathia. In: White NA, Moore JN, eds. Current Practice of Equine Surgery. Philadelphia: JB Lippincott, 1990.
19. Baker G. Diseases of teeth and paranasal sinuses. In: Colahan PT, Mayhew IG, Merritt AM, et al. eds. Equine Medicine and Surgery. 4th ed. Santa Barbara, CA: American Veterinary Publications, 1991:550.
20. DeBowes RM, Gaughan EM. Congenital dental disease of horses. Vet Clin North Am 1998;14:273–288.
21. Knottenbelt DC. The systemic effects of dental disease. In: Baker GJ, Easley J, eds. Equine Dentistry. Philadelphia: WB Saunders, 1999:136.

22. Knottenbelt DC. Oral and dental tumors. In: Baker GJ, Easley J, eds. Equine Dentistry. Philadelphia: WB Saunders, 1999:84–93.
23. Baker GJ. Abnormalities of development and eruption. In: Baker GJ, Easley J, eds. Equine Dentistry. Philadelphia: WB Saunders, 1999:59.
24. Knottenblet DC, Pascoe RR. Diseases and Disorders of the Horse. London: Wolfe Publishing, 1994:14.
25. Lingard DR, Crawford TB. Congenital ameloblastoma in a foal. Am J Vet Res 1970;31:801.
26. Roberts MC, Groenendyk S, Kelly WR. Ameloblastomic odontoma in a foal. Equine Vet 1978;10:91–93.
27. Lane JG, Gibbs C, Meynick SE, et al. Radiographic examination of the facial, nasal and paranasal sinus regions of the horse: I. Indications and procedures in 235 cases. Equine Vet J 1987;19:466–473.
28. Gibbs C, Lane JG. Radiographic examination of the facial, nasal and paranasal sinus regions of the horse: II. Radiologic findings. Equine Vet J 1987;19:474–482.
29. Morse CC, Saik JE, Richardson DW. Equine juvenile mandibular ossifying fibroma. Vet Pathol 1988;25:410–412.
30. Robbins SC, Arighi M, Ottewell G. The use of megavoltage radiation to treat juvenile mandibular ossifying fibroma in a horse. Can Vet J 1996;37:683–684.
31. Fessler JF. Heterotopic polydontia in horses: nine cases (1969-1986). J Am Vet Med Assoc 1988;192:535–538.
32. Goldstein G. The diagnosis and treatment of orthodontic problems. Probl Vet Med 1990;2:195–213.
33. Kertesz P. Orthodontics. In: Kertesz P, ed. A Color Atlas of Veterinary Dentistry and Oral Surgery. London: Wolfe Publishing 1993:63–72.
34. McIlwraith CW. Equine digestive system. In: Jennings PB, ed. The Practice of Large Animal Surgery. Philadelphia: WB Saunders, 1984:558–560.
35. Zetner K. Equine apicoectomy. In: Proceedings of the American Veterinary Dental College Meeting; New Orleans, LA 1989; pp. 104–105.
36. Emily PL. Equine orthodontics and endodontics. In: Proceedings of the Eastern States Veterinary Conference; Orlando, FL 1990; p. 148.

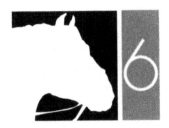

MATURE HORSE DENTISTRY

PATRICIA PENCE AND KRISTIN WILEWSKI

The horse is considered mature by its fifth birthday. By the age of 5, the horse should have shed all of its deciduous teeth; and the final set of permanent teeth, the corner incisors, should be coming into wear. Most breeds of horses have finished growing and have reached their adult size by their fifth year also. From this time on, the individual idiosyncrasies of skull conformation, the abnormalities of permanent tooth eruption, and the damage inflicted upon the dental unit by trauma will influence the manner in which the teeth are worn for the remainder of the horse's life.

The goal of equine dentistry is to recreate a functional masticatory unit if it strays from the ideal. This is accomplished by burring, filing, or cutting teeth that are too long and by balancing the chewing surfaces from side to side and front to back. Additionally, dentistry is used to remove any sources of oral discomfort for the horse, such as sharp enamel points, wolf teeth, and long, sharp canine teeth.

Mature horses are between 5 to 19 years of age. How often dentistry must be scheduled depends on the horse's dental conformation, diet, previous dental care (or lack of it), and level of performance. The higher the level of performance, the more frequently dentistry should be scheduled. Small dental problems can affect the efficiency of mastication and the horse's response to the rider's requests.

As a general rule, dentistry should be scheduled every 4 to 6 months for those horses that have teeth with occlusal areas not in wear and for those that are expected to perform at a high level. If the horse is young enough, and dentistry is scheduled often enough, many times the conformation that leads to overlong cheek teeth will stabilize after 2 years and future dentistry can be scheduled every 9 to 12 months (unless it is a high-level performance horse). Horses that have a full set of adult teeth, no orthodontic abnormalities, graze freely on pasture, and have low to nonexistent performance requirements may need dental care just once a year or even once every 2 years.

This chapter will discuss dentistry issues that are relevant to performance horses, as well as dental and oral abnormalities that are common in this age group.

■ ■   WOLF TEETH AND THE BITTED HORSE

Wolf teeth are vestiges of premolars that might have been functional in the horse millions of years ago but have no purpose now. Perhaps not all horses that have wolf teeth suffer from oral discomfort when bitted. However, considering that many horses endure a lot of oral pain without showing it, how are we to know which horses are suffering and which are not? Surely discomfort must be relative to the size and placement of the wolf teeth, the type and size of the bit, the amount of loose buccal mucosa in the individual horse, and the skill of the rider. The only way to know that the horse is as comfortable as possible is to remove the wolf teeth or reduce them to the gingival margin. See Chapter 11 for a description of wolf tooth extraction.

Anecdotal reports suggest that in many cases wolf teeth eventually ankylose to the bone as the horse gets older. It is not unusual to find wolf teeth that are broken at the alveolar margin and are attached only by the surrounding gingiva. These teeth are easily removed by elevating the gingival attachments and extracting the broken crown. The root is left in place. In the event that the tooth is not broken, it is less traumatic to the soft tissues and bone to grind or burr the crown of the wolf tooth level to the gingiva than it is to try to extract a large ankylosed tooth. Obviously, the approach to eliminating the pain caused by wolf teeth in a mature horse has to be analyzed on an individual basis.

■ ■   BIT SEATS: THEIR PURPOSE AND SHAPES

A *bit seat* is a term used to describe the rounded and smoothed rostral portion of the first cheek tooth.[1] Bit seats are referred to in the plural because they are a set of four rounded corners: the upper and lower right side and the upper and lower left side. Although all bitted horses should benefit from some degree of rounding off the rostral corners of the #06s, horses that wear snaffle bits will receive the greatest comfort. The headstalls of horses wearing a snaffle bit are usually adjusted until the bit lifts the commisures of the mouth into one to two wrinkles. The snaffle bit is jointed in the center and works partly by exerting pressure on the commisures of the mouth. The curb bit is "carried" in the mouth and is worn more rostrally. However, a sharp tug on a curb bit will create discomfort if the rostral cheek teeth are sharp and pointed.

The average horse that is usually ridden with a fairly loose rein (western pleasure, western equitation, and snaffle bit reining or cutting horses) probably gets the most benefit from the upper bit seats. Lower bit seats in horses ridden in this manner help prevent the occlusal surface of the lower tooth that is no longer in wear from overgrowing. Horses that are ridden with a lot of collection and/or a lot of contact with a snaffle bit (dressage horses, race horses, or harness horses) benefit from all four corner surfaces being round and smoothed because the commisures of the mouth, including the loose buccal mucosa, are drawn up into the bit at all times.

PRACTICE TIP:

Discomfort from wolf teeth and the sharp, right-angled corners on first upper cheek teeth is easy to appreciate if you try this exercise. Take your thumb and firmly press (or even jab) your own buccal gingiva into the tip of one of your own canine teeth. Now try to imagine that your canine tooth has a long, jagged edge on it, sharp enough to lacerate the inside of your cheek, and that someone else controls when you feel that pain and when you don't.

Just as there has always been controversy about whether to pull or not pull wolf teeth, there has been controversy about whether horses *need* bit seats. Try the above exercise if you don't think that rounding and smoothing the first cheek teeth would make a difference in the comfort of the horse.

The location of where to start the bevel of the bit seat is an area of equine dentistry that would benefit from a few simple controlled studies, which would end the arguments about it. One author suggests that the type of bit that the horse must carry may dictate the amount and angle of bevel.[2] This author says that for horses wearing a curb bit, the rounding of the corner should begin halfway up the exposed crown of the tooth. The bevel in horses wearing a snaffle bit should start at the level of the gingiva. Participants at the American Association of Equine Practitioners (AAEP) Dentistry Forum in 2001 made these comments: Narrow bits are more likely to pinch the buccal mucosa against the teeth. Horses wearing twisted wire snaffles or gag bits need more aggressive bit seats, i.e., more tooth will be taken out of occlusion. Aggressive bit seats should be created gradually to avoid entering the pulp. Horses with aggressive bit seats need to have them freshened up more often because sharp points form faster on the areas of the tooth that are taken out of occlusion.

Ideal bit seats address both the buccal and lingual (or palatal) surface of the tooth. They are smooth, polished, and symmetrical. Ideal bit seats blend invisibly into the occlusal surface. Techniques for creating bit seats are described in Chapter 4, Basic Dental Techniques.

KEY POINT:

▶ Do not create bit seats until you have corrected abnormalities in the first cheek teeth and have reestablished the table angles. A common mistake is to grind off a hook or the corner of a ramp without addressing the overall length of the tooth compared with the rest of the arcade. An overhanging upper tooth or ramped lower tooth that is still too long is just an abnormal tooth with a bit seat on it.

■ ■ **THE PERFORMANCE FLOAT**

The performance float is not a new concept. Even before power instruments were developed, there were veterinary and lay dentists who prided themselves on creating not only a functional dental unit, but one that provided the least distraction and the most comfort for elite equine athletes. With hand floats and files of different lengths and shapes, they molded bit seats and reduced the buccal enamel ridges. The finishing touches on the performance float are still mainly done by hand. Power instruments can be used to give the teeth their initial shape, but it requires skillful use of hand tools to give the tooth surfaces their final dressing.

Similar in concept to bit seats, the performance float dresses the buccal and lingual surfaces of the floated teeth. The buccal enamel ridges of the first three upper cheek teeth (#06, 07, and 08) receive the most critical attention. Starting at the gingival margin, the vertical enamel ridges (sulci) are smoothed even with the exposed crown. The sharp enamel points on the buccal corners of the occlusal surface are filed off, and the corners are rounded and blended from nonocclusal to occlusal crown. The nonocclusal surfaces on the palatal aspects of the upper teeth and the lingual aspects of the lower teeth are lightly dressed as needed to smooth rough areas. Finally, some practitioners put in what they call *caudal bit seats*. This is the process of rounding and dressing the caudal corners of the upper cheek teeth.

Canine teeth should be cut and smoothed. It is not necessary or even desirable to cut canines to the gingival margin. Cutting them too short will usually result in pulp exposure. In addition, it has been reported that some dressage judges will mark down horses whose tongues protrude from the sides of their mouths, which may occur if the corners are reduced too far.

KEY POINT:

▶ Before proceeding to the details of the performance float, all occlusal and conformation abnormalities must be corrected, and the table angles reestablished. The only dental procedure that does not need to be done before the performance float is the trimming and realigning of the incisors. The performance float puts a professional *polish* on cheek teeth that are already corrected and balanced.

■ ■ DENTAL ISSUES OF THE MATURE HORSE

History

Ask the owner or trainer if he or she has noticed any unusual eating patterns, such as holding the head in a peculiar manner while eating, chewing slowly and carefully, or chewing on just one side of the mouth. Does the horse eat for awhile, then stop and walk away dejectedly, taking a long time to eat? Does the horse take mouthfuls of hay over to the water trough and soak them before eating? Does the horse sometimes appear to have odd swellings in the cheeks that spontaneously appear and disappear? Does the caretaker of the horse find boluses of partially chewed food on the ground? Does the horse have problems maintaining or gaining weight, even if the portions of food are increased?

Also inquire whether the horse has any behavioral problems while being bridled or ridden. Horses that need expert dental care often exhibit some form of behavioral or performance problems. Many horse owners, even experienced performance horse trainers, do not associate behavioral problems or performance problems with dental pain. See *Box 6.1* for behavioral and performance problems that may be related to dental abnormalities.

Oral pain can keep any horse from performing to its full potential. A split-second lapse in concentration is all it takes to ruin a good run in timed events. A horse that is fussy with the bit, that keeps tossing out its nose and wringing its tail with irritation or anxiety will not show well in a pleasure class. A horse that will not accept the bit, bend its head nicely at the poll, and round its back for collected self-carriage will not show up to its potential in reining and dressage.

BOX 6.1 DENTAL-RELATED BEHAVIORAL AND PERFORMANCE PROBLEMS

Head tossing
Bit chewing
Refusal to carry the bit
Frequently trying to open the mouth
Reluctance to take a certain lead
Reluctance to bend at the poll or bend the neck
Running backwards
Going wide on turns
Not stopping squarely
Rearing
Unexplainable temper fits

Examination of the External Features of the Head

Examine the external features of the head. Look for abnormal swelling or draining tracts. Mentally divide the head in half on the sagittal midline. Compare one side with the other for symmetry of the muscles of mastication. Observe the ears to see if they are equally mobile. Examine the temporomandibular joints for symmetry, and palpate them to see if they are painful. Check the eyes to see if they are level with each other and the lids are equally functional. Check the lips to see if they droop to one side or the other. Palpate the ventral mandibles and interdental areas for swellings.

Check Lateral Excursion and Occlusion

Check lateral excursion by grasping the bridge of the nose with one hand and the ventral mandible with the other. Move the mandible side to side and listen carefully to the sounds or lack of sounds emanating from the caudal cheek teeth, rostral cheek teeth, and incisors. Feel to see if the jaw is moving freely, or if it locks up on one side or the other. Lack of free movement is a sign that there are overgrown teeth.

Soft-Tissue Trauma

After examining the outer features of the head, sedate the horse and apply a full-mouth speculum. Examine all the mucosal surfaces, the tongue, and the hard palate. Record oral abnormalities in the dental chart. Look for lacerations to the tongue and buccal mucosa (*Figs. 6.1 and 6.2*). The buccal mucosa of horses that have endured years of sharp enamel points will be discolored and calloused (*Fig. 6.3*). In extreme cases, the callous may be thick and wrinkled from chronic abrasion. Check the mucosa opposite the upper #11 cheek teeth. The cheek skin is tighter there, and many horses have a callus or even an ulcer in that area. Examine the hard palate for signs of injury from high port bits. Palpate the interdental area (the bars) for blind wolf teeth, unerupted canine teeth, and bone spurs caused by biting injuries.

Apical Infections

Tooth root infections are not uncommon in the mature horse. Infections of the apical area may be secondary to dental caries, hypoplastic infundibula, periodontal disease, and direct access of bacteria to the tooth pulp due to trauma.[3–5] In the mature horse, infection of the maxillary cheek teeth is more common than infection of the mandibular cheek teeth.[5,6]

Although uncommon in horses over the age of 5 years, clinical signs of mandibular tooth root infections include swelling in the apical region of the affected tooth, fistula formation, and foul breath if the infection drains into the mouth.[4]

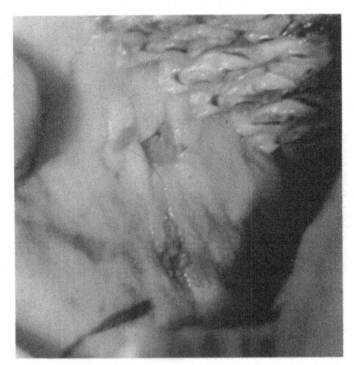

Figure 6.1 Severe trauma to the buccal mucosa caused by the use of a tight cavesson to keep the mouth shut in a horse that has extremely long maxillary enamel points. (Photograph used with permission from Proper Equine Dentistry by Tony Basile, 2000, CD-ROM.)

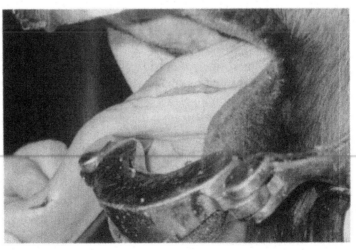

Figure 6.2 Healing laceration to the lateral edge of the tongue caused by long enamel points on mandibular teeth.

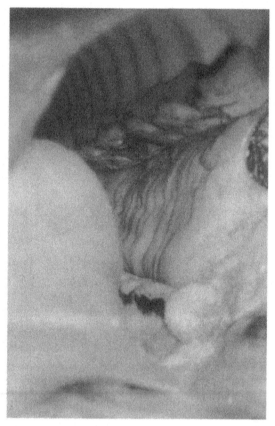

Figure 6.3 Calloused and discolored buccal mucosa caused by years of chronic irritation from long enamel points.

Clinical signs of maxillary tooth root infection depend on which tooth is affected.[4] The first two maxillary teeth (#06 and 07) do not lie within any sinus structures. Infection involving these teeth may appear as facial swelling, a draining fistulous tract, or foul breath if the purulent exudate drains into the mouth. Tooth roots of maxillary cheek teeth #08, 09, and 10 lie within the rostral maxillary sinus and those of #11 lie within the caudal maxillary sinus. Infection involving these teeth will destroy the alveolar bone overlying the tooth root, allowing exudate to enter the sinus. A thick, foul-smelling nasal discharge, unilateral if only one side is involved, may appear from the ipsilateral nostril. Percussing the sinus will elicit a dull sound compared with the hollow sound of a normal sinus. Long-standing infections involving a sinus may deform the facial bones and the airway on that side of the face, creating inspiratory dyspnea.[7] Infections involving the nasolacrimal duct may result in ocular drainage.

Radiographic signs of apical disease include alveolar bone lysis, lysis of surrounding bone with or without fistulation, lysis of the tooth root, and sclerosis of bone in the infected area.[8–10] Oblique radiographic views taken with the cassette placed on the side of the affected teeth will give the clearest images. Lateral views in the standing horse may show a fluid line if there is fluid in the sinus.

Treatment of infection of the maxillary cheek teeth in which loss of periodontal structures is evident is usually limited to extraction of the affected tooth. The complexity of the root and pulp canals makes endodontic treatment very difficult. As of this writing, the results are better in mandibular teeth than in maxillary teeth.[11]

Periodontal Disease

Check the interproximal spaces on both the lingual and buccal sides for signs of food impacted between the teeth, gingivitis, and periodontal pockets. A dental mirror or endoscope will be needed to examine the buccal aspects of the caudal cheek teeth. Horses with severe periodontal disease may quid their food and develop secondary dental malocclusions from abnormal mastication.[12] For more information, see Chapter 10, Dental Infections.

Dental Decay

Look for dental caries. Caries are focal areas of demineralization of the teeth. Caries on the incisors appear as areas in which the cemental layer is gone and the underlying enamel appears blackened. Check for pitting of the infundibula of the maxillary teeth, a sign of hypoplastic cemental lakes. Clean out any food-packed infundibula, and assess whether caries are present. Infundibular caries have been reported in up to 43% of horses that have otherwise normal teeth.[3] Caries begin as brown or black areas in the cemental lakes. As the degenerative process continues, the lesion becomes deeper and begins to involve the enamel, which also darkens in color. Advanced lesions have deep pitting of the infundibulae, some of which coalesce due to degeneration of the enamel separating them. Unless the caries invade the pulp or result in the fracture of the tooth, horses do not usually show clinical signs related to this condition. For more information on caries, see Chapter 10, Dental Infections.

Fractured Teeth

The dental examination may reveal a tooth with part of the crown missing because it was fractured off. Further investigation is needed if the fracture involves more than an insignificant portion of the crown and if it extends below the gingival margin. A radiographic examination may help to determine the condition of the tooth root. If the tooth is split down the middle with the center of the tooth exposed, and the fracture is more than a few hours old, the tooth will have to eventually be extracted because the pulp will invariably be infected. If only a piece of the crown is missing and the remainder of the tooth is healthy, the tooth should be left alone. Periodic dressing of the opposing tooth may be necessary if it grows into the missing area of the occlusal surface.

Absent Cheek Teeth and Diastema (See Step Mouth)

Diastema

Diastema are interproximal spaces between teeth. In a long-term study of 400 cases, Dixon et al. found that diastema were the primary dental disorder in 16 horses.[12] The diastema occurred in both the mandibular and maxillary arcades with equal frequency and were most commonly present between the caudal cheek teeth, especially between teeth #09 and 10. Food impaction in the interproximal spaces led to periodontal pocketing that eventually spread to both the lateral and medial margins of

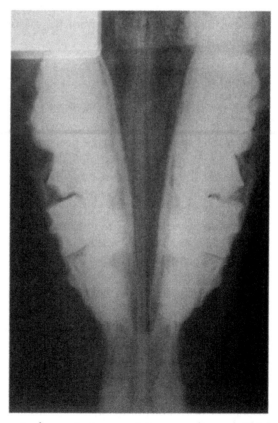

Figure 6.4   Diastema is often easier to appreciate on a radiograph. This horse has twisted and displaced maxillary #08s due to overcrowding.

the adjacent teeth. Clinical signs included severe, chronic quidding, attributed to oral pain caused by the extensive periodontal disease, dental sinusitis, and apical infections. Dental overgrowths were present in 10 of the 16 horses and were also attributed to abnormal occlusive movements caused by pain secondary to severe periodontal disease.

Both developmental and acquired diastema have been described.[12] Developmental diastema were attributed to abnormally wide embryonic development of dental buds and to abnormal eruption of permanent teeth. Teeth that erupted laterally or medially to the rest of the arcade or that erupted in a twisted manner frequently have diastema between adjacent teeth *(Fig. 6.4)*. Although severe periodontal disease is not common in young horses, developmental diastema was found to cause periodontal disease in horses less than 5 years of age in this study.

Acquired diastema occur when dental disease results in loose and abnormally positioned teeth or the loss of teeth.[12] It was noted that there is an increasing tendency for diastema to develop as horses age *(Fig. 6.5)*. The presence of the large interdental space between the cheek teeth and the incisors disrupts the continuity of the dental arch. Insufficient caudal angulation of the crown of the first cheek teeth (the #06s) and/or insufficient rostral angulation of the last cheek teeth (the #11s) that results in inadequate compression of the teeth was proposed to be the cause of diastema in some cases.

At this time, there is no practical way to correct the diastema in and of themselves. Treatment revolves around correcting occlusal abnormalities, extraction of

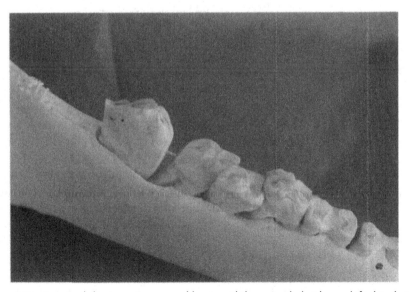

Figure 6.5 Acquired diastema in an aged horse with loose teeth that have shifted in their alveolar sockets.

diseased teeth, and frequent cleaning out of periodontal pockets.[12] Five of the 16 horses in the Dixon study were euthanized due to the severity of periodontal disease or poor response to treatment.

Supernumerary Teeth

Supernumerary teeth are not common and are thought to be associated with splitting of the tooth bud.[13] Malocclusions can be created by overcrowding, especially in the cheek teeth. Supernumerary incisors may not result in overcrowding because of the extra space for teeth to spread out in the interdental area. Teeth that are not in occlusion will need frequent reduction to prevent soft-tissue damage due to overgrowth. See Displaced Cheek Teeth for further discussion of the effects of supernumerary teeth.

Displaced Cheek Teeth

Displaced cheek teeth can originate as developmental displacements or acquired displacements. Developmental displacements occur during the period of eruption of permanent teeth. Overcrowding, due to delayed eruption of a tooth, is the primary source of displacements and is frequently bilateral.[12] This condition is more common in horses with small heads, especially ponies, miniature horses, and Arabians. Supernumerary cheek teeth can also create overcrowding. If the displacement results in occlusal surfaces that are not in wear, overgrowths may be present. Long overgrowths are an indication that the displacements are long-standing. Occasionally, displaced teeth are slightly rotated instead of aligned with the adjacent teeth (Fig. 6.5). Clinical signs include quidding, trauma to the tongue or cheeks, refusal to carry the bit, and abnormal head carriage. Large spaces may be present if there is incomplete contact between adjacent teeth. Food accumulates in these gaps, leading to gingivitis and periodontal disease.

Developmental displacements are seen most commonly in the caudal three-cheek teeth.[12] Premolars can be affected if the deciduous tooth is lost prematurely, before the permanent tooth completely fills the subgingival space between adjacent permanent teeth. The result is a partial closure of the space in which the permanent tooth needed to erupt into, causing the tooth to erupt off its mark.[14]

Acquired displacements are usually seen in older horses. Relatively normal occlusal wear is an indication that the displacement is relatively recent.[12] Acquired displacements may be caused by years of abnormal occlusal forces applied to just one side of the tooth or by the tooth becoming loose in its alveolar socket (*Fig. 6.6*). If periodontal disease invades the alveolar socket, the periodontal attachments will eventually be broken. Loss of periodontal tissues leaves more room for the tooth to move in the alveolus. The most common acquired displacement of maxillary teeth is the palatal displacement of the last molars (the #11s).[12]

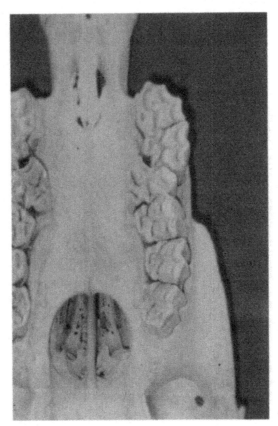

Figure 6.6 Malformed, rotated, and displaced cheek teeth caused by severe overcrowding in this miniature horse.

Severely displaced teeth with no occlusal contact and displaced teeth with that are associated with extensive periodontal disease should be extracted. Extraction may also be indicated if severe quidding of food continues after more conservative treatment.[12]

Less severely displaced teeth require removal of large overgrowths by cutting or grinding them off. Smaller overgrowths can be rasped off.

Abnormalities of Wear

Hooks and Ramps. Hooks on the upper #06s or lower #11s and ramps on the lower #06s are very common abnormalities that interfere with mastication and greatly affect the comfort of the performance horse *(Figs. 6.7, 6.8, 6.9)*. These cause a block in the lateral excursion that can sometimes be detected when moving the mandible from side to side. These abnormalities also put pressure on the temporomandibular

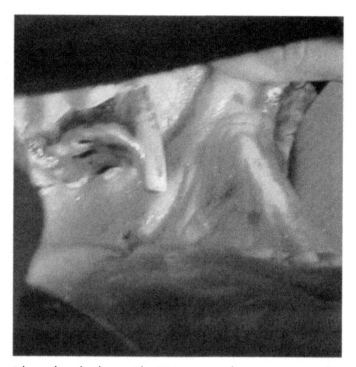

Figure 6.7   A long, sharp hook on tooth #106 can cause horses to resent and avoid the bit because the bit pinches the loose buccal mucosa against the hook. (Photograph used with permission from Proper Equine Dentistry by Tony Basile, 2000, CD-ROM.)

joint (TMJ), which is another source of performance and mastication problems. Lower #06 ramps tend to force the mandible rostrally, and rostral upper #06 hooks with caudal lower #11 hooks tend to force the mandible caudally. Horses with this conformation may resist collection because the head carriage required by collection causes the mandible to move rostrally, which increases pressure on the overlong teeth and the TMJ. Horses with rostral hooks on the upper #06s may also react by rearing up when pressure is applied to the bit. Caudal pressure on the bit pinches the commissures of the lips under the point of the hook. These hooks become more pronounced over time and need to be attended to at each dental procedure.

Treatment involves reducing the overlong portion of the tooth. In the case of large, long hooks, it is possible to create an area of pulpal exposure 1 to 3 mm in diameter. Either be prepared to sterilize and apply a thin cap to such a tooth, or don't remove all of it at once. Remove most of the bulk of the hook, but do not keep removing tooth material to level a large hook at the first appointment. Waiting 3 to 4 months will allow sufficient secondary dentin formation to protect the pulp. In horses older than 15 years, do not completely level large ramps on upper or lower #06s because anecdotal reports suggest the opposing tooth won't erupt fast enough

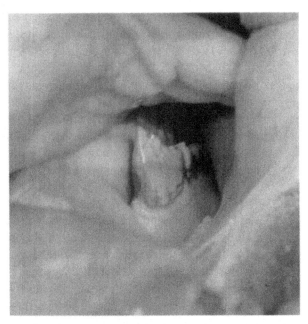

Figure 6.8 This is referred to as a ramp malocclusion. The opposing tooth was excessively short compared with the rest of the arcade. (Photograph used with permission from Proper Equine Dentistry by Tony Basile, 2000, CD-ROM.)

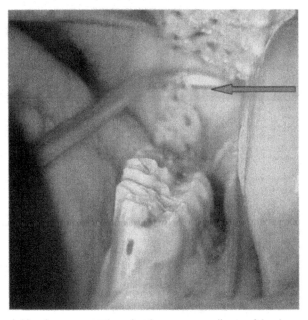

Figure 6.9 Caudal hook on #411. These hooks are especially painful in horses that are asked to bend at the poll. Caudal hooks can erupt long enough to lacerate the palatine artery. (Photograph used with permission from Proper Equine Dentistry by Tony Basile, 2000, CD-ROM.)

for those teeth to ever be in occlusion again. Regarding caudal hooks and ramps, be sure there truly is an overlong area and not just the illusion created by the curvature of the jaw (see Chapter 4, Basic Dental Techniques).

Wave Mouth. *Wave mouth* is an abnormality in which there is an undulating occlusal surface in which several teeth are involved *(Fig. 6.10)*. This condition is common and tends to become more pronounced if not corrected each time the teeth are floated. Early in the condition, it may be easier to palpate the unevenness of the arcade than it is to see it. Wave mouth may be present in both sides of the mouth, or it may be more prominent on one side.

The etiology of wave mouth is not known, but several factors may be involved *(Box 6.2)*. This is an area of dentistry that would benefit from further study.

A common presentation is for one to three cheek teeth in the middle of the lower arcade to be longer than the other teeth in the arcade. The opposing teeth in the upper arcade will be shorter than the other teeth in the upper arcade. Variations include a wave with hooks or ramps on either the upper or lower rostral #06s and a wave with long upper #10s. Occasionally, they may have long lower #06s, upper #07s, lower #08s, upper #10s, and lower #11s. The wave may involve more than one tooth, such

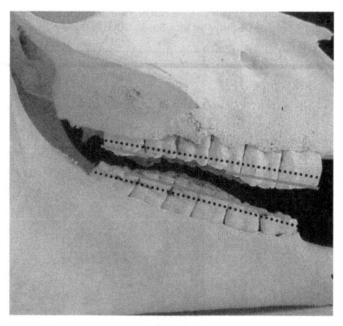

Figure 6.10   This horse has a bilateral 8-9-10 wave malocclusion. In addition, the upper #06s, 07s, and 10s are too long. The solid lines show what should be reduced and the dotted lines approximate where the gingival margin would be in the living horse. (Photograph used with permission from Proper Equine Dentistry by Tony Basile, 2000, CD-ROM.)

BOX 6.2 FACTORS THAT MAY PLAY A ROLE IN CREATING A WAVE CONFORMATION

1. Different rates of eruption may occur in these teeth due to asynchronous shedding of deciduous teeth.
2. Loss of periodontal fibers due to periodontal disease may delay eruption of affected teeth.[15]
3. The loss of tooth substance to infundibular caries of the maxillary teeth may predispose them to increased wear.[16]
4. Mechanical forces exerted on the static maxillary cheek teeth by the mobile mandibular teeth could create localized tooth loss of the maxillary cheek teeth.[15]

---

as the caudal half of the lower #07s, the entire #08s, the rostral half of the lower #09s, or the rostral half of the upper #09s, the entire upper #10s, and the rostral half of the upper #11s. In the horse with a subtle wave mouth, the overlong teeth may simply have a flat table angle, rather than the entire tooth being long. This is more common on the upper #10s, but may be seen on any tooth. This condition can be easily corrected by recreating the appropriate table angle with a few rubs of an S file.

Treatment for correcting wave mouth depends on its severity, the length of the incisors, and the age of the horse. Total correction of wave mouth is possible to do in one dentistry appointment, but there are several important issues to consider. The shortest teeth in the mouth must be long enough to level the mouth to, without getting into pulp on the longest teeth. The incisors must be long enough so they can be trimmed down to get the cheek teeth back into occlusion. To meet these conditions, the longest teeth in the wave should not need to have more than approximately 4 mm of tooth removed. The incisors must have enough crown exposed beyond the gingival margin so that you will not have to reduce them to the gingival margin. Anecdotal reports suggest that the pulp is closer to the incisal surface in the lower incisors than it is in the upper incisors, so it is usually difficult to remove more than 1.5 to 2 mm off the lower incisors without causing the horse extreme discomfort.

It is best to do the correction over a period of time in horses that have severe wave conditions and in horses that are older than approximately 15 years of age.[15] Anecdotal reports suggest that to totally flatten the tallest portion of a severe wave in a horse older than 15 years may take those teeth out of occlusion for the remainder of the horse's life, because the opposing teeth may not erupt fast enough to fill in the gap. In a younger horse, this will help prevent taking the mouth totally out of occlusion because the incisors can't be cut down enough. Severe waves should be worked on about every 6 months until the wave is corrected. This can take 1 to 2 years.

Exaggerated Transverse Ridges (ETRs). Normal cheek teeth have transverse ridges on their occlusal surfaces created by the folding of the enamel *(Fig. 6.11)*. The occlusal ridges are arranged in an attenuated sawtooth pattern in which the maxillary and mandibular ridges compliment each other, creating a surface conducive to shearing roughages. However, some mastication patterns may encourage this ridging to become so exaggerated that the maxilla and the mandible interlock, thus inhibiting the rostral/caudal movement of the mandible that is necessary when the jaws are in neutral position and the horse is asked to bend at the poll *(Fig. 6.12)*. Treatment involves returning the ridges to their attenuated form by burring or filing off the longest parts of the *sawtooth*, without completely flattening the occlusal surface or changing the table angle.

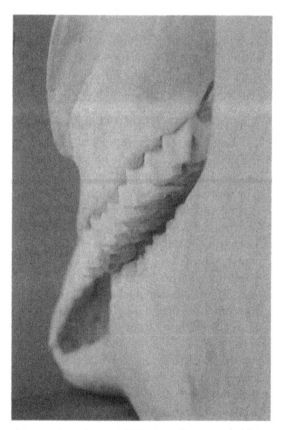

Figure 6.11 Normal transverse ridges are difficult to illustrate in a photograph. This young horse has transverse wave on the occlusal surface of the cheek teeth that are long enough to shred roughage, but not so long that rostral–caudal motion is inhibited. This view also illustrates how the enamel folding can result in deep buccal ridges.

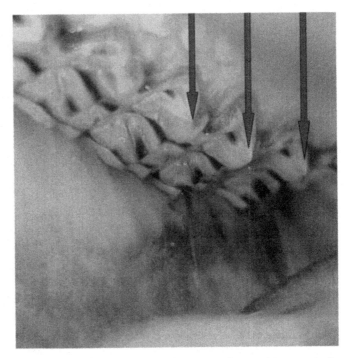

Figure 6.12 It is easy to see how excessive transverse ridges such as seen in the caudal cheek teeth of this horse could interlock with ridges on the opposing teeth, and prevent rostral–caudal movement of the mandible. (Photograph used with permission from Proper Equine Dentistry by Tony Basile, 2000, CD-ROM.)

Step Mouth. Teeth may be absent due to a congenital defect in which the tooth bud is absent, because of trauma or to periapical infection and subsequent extraction. Absent cheek teeth cause severe dental problems if not addressed on a regular basis *(Fig. 6.13)*. The occlusal surface in the opposite arcade, usually the caudal surface of one tooth and the rostral surface of an adjacent tooth, will grow into the gap. The arcade in which the tooth is missing will also be affected. The loss of a tooth disrupts the stability of the arcade. The lack of opposing pressure allows the adjacent teeth to drift toward the gap. This results in a gap (or gaps) down the line in other locations in the arcade. These gaps become packed with food. Eventually, severe periodontal disease will be associated with the gingival areas that are inflamed from the fermented food packed into the periodontal pockets.

The occlusal surface of teeth opposite the missing tooth will have to be reduced every 6 to 12 months. The author (Wilewski) has had some success applying acrylic patches into the gap. See Case Report #3.

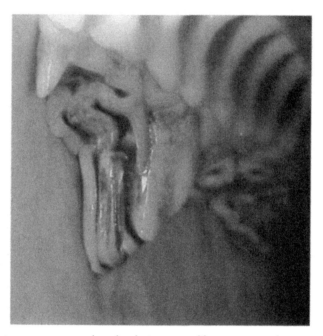

Figure 6.13 A severe step-mouth malocclusion caused by missing tooth #407. Notice how the caudal portion of tooth #106 and the rostral portion of tooth #107 have erupted into the space. In addition, a hook is present on #106. (Photograph used with permission from Proper Equine Dentistry by Tony Basile, 2000, CD-ROM.)

Shear Mouth. Shear mouth can be defined as an arcade in which the occlusal surface greatly exceeds 15 degrees of angulation. The buccal side of the maxillary teeth is extremely long and the lingual side of the maxillary teeth is very short, sometimes worn to the gingival surface. The mandibular teeth are the mirror image of the maxillary teeth, with an excessively long lingual side and a very short buccal side. Shear mouth may be unilateral or bilateral.

Unilateral shear mouth can be secondary to the traumatic medial displacement of the right or left hemimandible. See Case Report #4.

Incisor Malocclusions. Incisor malocclusions may be developmental or acquired. Developmental malocclusions, such as parrot-mouth and sow-mouth, are described in detail in Chapter 5. These malocclusions cannot be corrected in the mature horse, but will need yearly or biyearly corrective dentistry to address the continuous growth of areas of the teeth that are not in occlusion. The incisors will need to be kept short enough so that they do not interfere with lateral excursion. Free up the mandible by removing any hooks or ramps that may be present on the cheek teeth.

Slant bite, ventral curvature, and dorsal curvature are acquired incisor malocclusions. Slant bite may or may not be accompanied by abnormalities in the cheek teeth. Abnormal mastication due to unilateral dental abnormalities or disease may be responsible for some cases of slant bite and need to be corrected.

Ventral curvature (smile conformation) is most commonly seen in older mature horses and appears to be associated with the increase in angulation of the incisors. Whether this is a pathological condition and how much correction needs to be done is debatable at this time. It would seem reasonable that some correction may be needed if lateral excursion is impaired or if there is an acquired overjet of the central pairs of incisors associated with the ventral curvature.

Dorsal curvature (frown conformation) is seen less often than slant or ventral curvature in the authors' experience. Dorsal curvature may be associated with cribbing.

Step-bite may be a developmental or acquired incisor malocclusion in which an irregularly uneven incisal surface is present. Lack of eruption of permanent incisors due to lack of embryonic tissue is uncommon and would be an abnormality that is developmental in nature. Maleruptions in which occlusion is impaired can be developmental or acquired. Acquired step-bite is commonly related to injury to either erupted or unerupted permanent incisors. Injury to unerupted permanent teeth may result in the deformity or abnormal position of the tooth. Injury to the erupted tooth may result in a transverse fracture of the tooth crown or an apical infection and subsequent loss of the tooth.

Neoplasia

Tumors of dental origin are relatively uncommon in the horse. Most of these tumors are not malignant, but they are locally invasive and may grow to such a large size that by the time they are recognized, management is difficult. Tumors of the paranasal sinuses, by contrast, are more often malignant than not. Oral or dental tumors are typically more common in young horses than in older ones. Because many oral tumors look the same, definitive diagnosis often depends on histological examination. There are many different neoplasms that may be seen in the mouth or head region. Listed below are a few of the more common ones.

Oral and dental neoplasms of the mature horse can involve tissues of the teeth (odontogenic tumors), bone (osteogenic tumors), or soft tissues.

Odontogenic tumors can occur in horses of any age. The most common odontogenic tumor of the mature horse is the ameloblastoma.[18] These are benign but locally invasive tumors, usually found in the mandible of older horses. Ameloblastomas are firm, well-demarcated tumors that are expansive rather than destructive. These masses contain no dentin or enamel. This differentiates them from the ameloblastic odontomas usually seen in the maxillary region of younger horses, which do contain dental elements.[19]

Another group of odontogenic tumors that may be seen in horses in this age group are complex and compound odontomas.[20] Both of these tumors contain all the elements of a normal tooth. In the complex odontoma, the dental elements are not organized. In the compound odontoma, the dental elements may look somewhat tooth-like.

Osteogenic tumors are rare in the horse. Osteosarcomas are malignant bone tumors that are usually seen in the mandible. Osteomas are benign, slow-growing tumors. They are reported to occur more often in the mandible than the maxilla.[21]

Squamous cell carcinomas are malignant, aggressive soft-tissue neoplasms that may be seen inside the mouth, inside the paranasal sinuses, and at the mucocutaneous junctions of the lips.[21–23] These tumors are typically slow growing, invasive, and destructive.[21,22]

Melanomas are tumors of melanocytes seen in mature, gray horses. Commonly seen in other areas of the body, particularly the anus, tail, and perineal region, they may also be found in the commisures of the lips, at the base of the ears, and in the parotid gland regions.[24]

Sarcoids are fibroblastic tumors of the skin. The nodular form of sarcoid may be found in the commisure of the lips.[25]

Treatment of oral and dental tumors is beyond the scope of this book and has been described elsewhere.[26–29]

■ ■   **CASE REPORTS**

All cases and photographs were provided by Kristin Wilewski.

Case Report #1 *(Figs. 6.14A, B)*

This is a 13-year-old Thoroughbred hunter-jumper gelding that apparently suffered trauma to the upper incisors at a young age. The permanent #101 and 102 never fully developed, allowing the permanent #401 and 402 to become severely overgrown. This created an obvious block to lateral excursion and, not surprisingly, this gelding was a very sloppy eater. The rider also found this horse to be resistant to turning commands. The molar arcades had only minor abnormalities—a ramped #306 and 406 and sharp enamel points. The ramps were reduced by burring, the arcades were floated, and bit seats were created. After the molar work was finished, the incisors were realigned to allow this horse full use of his mandible. The gingival margin had followed the overlong #401 and 402 and had to be resected as these teeth were reduced.

After this dental, this horse was able to chew his feed properly without losing it, and he became much more responsive to his rider's cues. Future dentals were scheduled every 6 months. Figures 6-14A and B show his incisors before and after the dentistry.

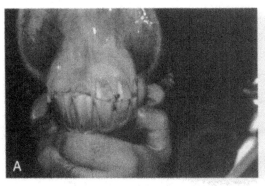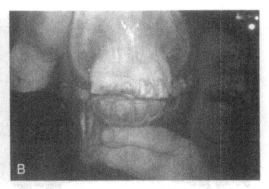

Figure 6.14 **A.** Trauma to the premaxilla and incisors as a young horse are the most likely cause of the dental problems in this horse. The permanent #101 and #102 never fully developed, allowing the #401 and #402 to overgrow and cause an obvious block to normal chewing motion. **B.** This is the same horse after a full dental, including incisor bite realignment. Teeth #401 and #402 had to be reduced to below the gingival margin to achieve proper balance and to ensure no interference from these teeth as they erupt again. Although the pulp cavity was exposed in #401 and #402, no complications ensued.

Case Report #2 *(Figs. 6.15A–G)*

This is a 10-year-old Appaloosa gelding used for pleasure riding and 4-H shows. He had a wave mouth conformation that was worse on the right side with rostral and caudal hooks, sharp enamel points, and slanted incisors. The overlong or hooked #106, 110, 206, 210, 308, 311, and 408 were burred level. The #411 hook was cut with C-head molar cutters, then smoothed, and the table angle was restored by burring. All arcades were floated, and the table angles were restored. Bit seats were created. Finally, the incisors were realigned to correct the slant bite and reduced until good molar occlusion was achieved. Figures 6.15A–G show his mouth before and after the dentistry.

Case Report #3 *(Figs. 6.16A, B)*

This case is unusual. It involved a 6-year-old Hackney Pony gelding that was performing at a high level in competition. During the initial examination, an unusual wave mouth conformation was discovered. The #108 and 208 were overlong (Fig. 6.16A). On closer inspection, the #308 and 408 were found to be very short and malodorous. At this visit, the wave was corrected by reducing the overlong #108 and 208 until they were level with their corresponding arcades. All arcades were floated and bit seats were created.

Radiographs were made to determine the status of the #308 and 408. The radiographs revealed the absence of permanent #308 and 408 (Fig. 6.16A and B). The

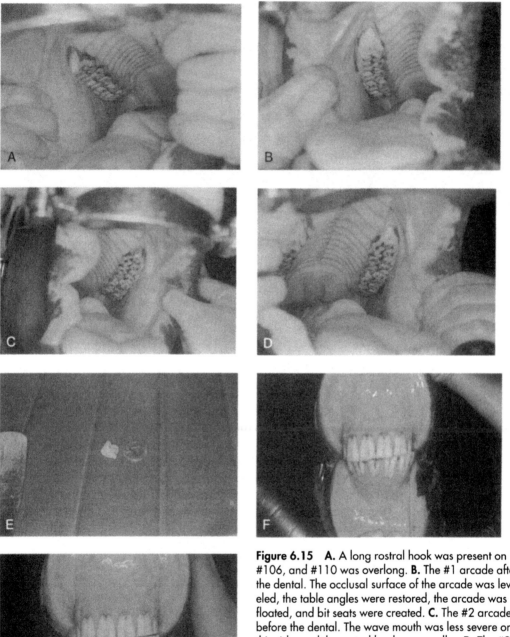

Figure 6.15 A. A long rostral hook was present on #106, and #110 was overlong. **B.** The #1 arcade after the dental. The occlusal surface of the arcade was leveled, the table angles were restored, the arcade was floated, and bit seats were created. **C.** The #2 arcade before the dental. The wave mouth was less severe on this side, and the rostral hook was smaller. **D.** The #2 arcade after the dental. **E.** The #411 hook that was cut off with molar cutters. **F.** The incisors before realignment. Notice the slant bite. **G.** The incisors after realignment. The lower incisors are shifted to the left, causing the neutral position to be off center. This could be due to a congenital defect or to a malalignment of the temporomandibular joint.

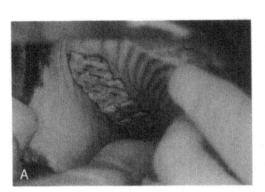 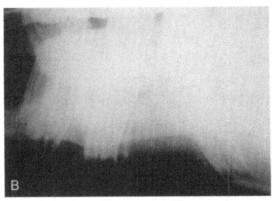

Figure 6.16 **A.** An unusual mouth conformation in which the #108 and #208 were overlong. **B.** Oblique radiographic views of the mandible show that there was no permanent #308 or #408.

tooth structures seen in the mouth were remnants of deciduous teeth that were quickly disintegrating.

After the show season was over, these fragments of the deciduous teeth were removed and the soft tissue was allowed to heal. Acrylic patches were formed into the shape of the missing teeth and placed into the gaps. The acrylic patch served to prevent the drifting of the remaining teeth into the spaces left by the deciduous teeth. The patches were rechecked every 6 months and changed as needed. Corrective dentistry will be needed for this pony for the rest of its life to prevent overgrowth of #108 and 208.

Case Report #4 *(Figs. 6.17A–E)*

This is a 13-year-old Trakahner broodmare with a shear mouth conformation on the right side of the mouth. The corrective dentistry performed on this mare included cutting the abnormal cheek teeth on the right side with B-, C-, and D-molar cutters, depending on the amount and size of tooth that needed cutting. Some teeth did not cut well because of the severe angle of the shear. Before using the cutters, the most rostral tooth to the tooth that was to be cut was burred until the cutters could be positioned. After the overlong teeth were reduced, a correct table angle was created using a burr. Twelve cheek teeth (six upper and six lower) had to be cut and burred.

Abnormalities on the left side of this mare's mouth included a hook on #206 and a long #308. Both of these problems were corrected by burring, and the table angles were reestablished. All arcades were floated. Bit seats were not necessary.

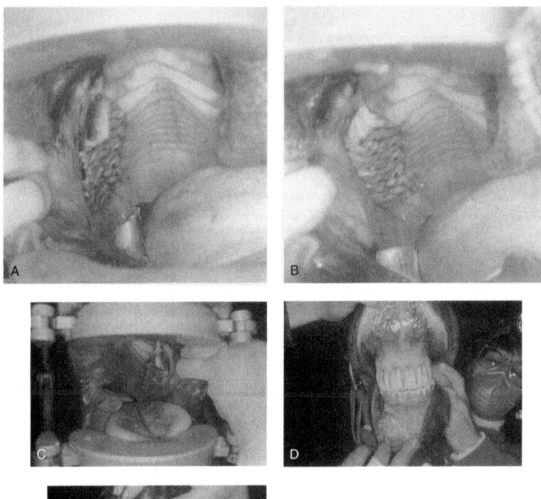

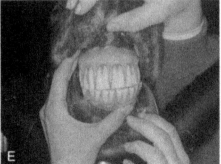

Figure 6.17   A. Shear mouth of the right side of the mouth (#1 and #4 arcades). **B.** Right side of the mouth after cutting and burring to reduce the shear mouth and correct the table angles. **C.** The incisors had a slight slant bite, but the mare carried her mandible to the left, which suggests an abnormality of the temporomandibular joint. **D.** The incisors after realignment. **E.** The mare still carries her mandible to the left.

The incisors had a slight slant bite. Very little reduction had to be done on the incisors to obtain good occlusion on the left side. After this dental work, the mare still had very limited mobility of the mandible to the right. This was probably due to a deformed TMJ. That there was a problem with the TMJ was also suggested by the tendency of this mare to carry her lower jaw to the left side, both before and after the incisor bite realignment. Figures 6.17A–E show this mare before and after the dentistry.

■ ■ REFERENCES

1. Wilewski KA, Rubin L. Bit seats: a dental procedure for enhancing performance of show horses. Equine Practice 1999;21:16.
2. Scrutchfield WL. Dental prophylaxis. In: Baker GJ, Easley J, eds. Equine dentistry. Philadelphia: WB Saunders, 1999:190–192.
3. Baker GJ. Some aspects of equine dental decay. Equine Vet J 1974;(6):127–130.
4. Baker GJ. Dental decay and endodontic disease. In: Baker GJ, Easley J, eds. Equine dentistry. Philadelphia: WB Saunders, 1999:79–84.
5. Dixon PM, Tremaine WH, Pickles K, Kuhns L, et al. Equine dental disease part 4: a long-term study of 400 cases: apical infections of cheek teeth. Equine Vet J 2000;32(3)182–194.
6. Prichard MA, Hacket R, Erb HN. Long-term outcome of tooth repulsion in horses, a retrospective of 61 Cases. Vet Surg 1992;21:145.
7. Hennig GE, Steckel RR. Diseases of the oral cavity and esophagus. In: Kobluk CN, Ames TR, Geor RJ, eds. The Horse: Diseases & Clinical Management. Philadelphia: WB Saunders, 1995:290–293.
8. Baker GJ. Some aspects of equine dental radiology. Equine Vet J 1971;3:46–51.
9. Gibbs C, Lane JG. Radiographic examination of the facial, nasal and paranasal sinus regions of the horse. II. Radiological findings. Equine Vet J 1987;19:474–482.
10. Park RD. Radiographic examination of the equine head. Vet Clin North Am Equine Pract 1993:9:49–74.
11. Baker GJ, Kirkland DK. Endodontic therapy in the horse. Proceedings of the 38th annual meeting of the American Association of Equine Practitioners, 1992:329–335.
12. Dixon PM, Tremaine WH, Pickles K, Kuhns L, et al. Equine dental disease part 2: a long-term study of 400 cases: disorders of development and eruption and variations in position of the cheek teeth. Equine Vet J 1999;31:519–528.
13. Baker GJ. Diseases of the teeth. In: Colahan PT, Mayhew IG, Merritt AM, eds. Equine Medicine and Surgery. 4th ed. Santa Barbara, CA: American Veterinary Publications, 1991.
14. Miles AEW, Grigson C. Colyer's Variation and Diseases of the Teeth of Animals. Revised ed. Cambridge, UK: Cambridge University Press, 1990:118–122.
15. Dixon PM, Tremaine WH, Pickles K, Kuhns L, et al. Equine dental disease part 3: a long-term study of 400 cases: disorders of wear, traumatic damage and idiopathic fractures, tumours and miscellaneous disorders of the cheek teeth. Equine Vet J 2000;32:9–18.
16. Easley J. Dental corrective procedures. Vet Clin North Am Equine Pract 1998;14: 411–432.

17. Knottenbelt DC. Oral and dental tumors. In: Baker GJ, Easley J, eds. Equine Dentistry. Philadelphia: WB Saunders, 1999:85–103.

18. Hanselka DW, Roberts RE, Thompson RB. Adamantinoma of the equine mandible. Vet Med Small Anim Clinician 1974;69:157–160.

19. Pirie RS, Dixon PM. Mandibular tumors in the horse: a review of the literature and seven case reports. Equine Vet Educ 1993;5:287–294.

20. Dubielzig RR, Beck KA, Levine S, Wilson JW. Complex odontoma in a stallion. Vet Pathol 1986;23:633–635.

21. Pool RR. Tumours of bone and cartilage. In: Moulton J, ed. Tumours in Domestic Animals. 3rd ed. Berkeley: University of California Press, 1990:157.

22. Thorp F, Graham R. A large osteosarcoma of the mandible. J Am Vet Med Assoc 1934;84:118–119.

23. Strafuss AC. Squamous cell carcinoma in horses. J Am Vet Med Assoc 1976;168:61–62.

24. Howie F, Munroe G, Thompson H, Murphy D. Palatine squamous cell carcinoma involving the maxillary sinus in two horses. Equine Vet Educ 1992;4:3–7.

25. Goetz TE, Long MT. Treatment of melanoma in horses. Compend of Contin Educ 1993;15:608–610.

26. Knottenbelt DC, Edwards SER, Daniel EA. The diagnosis and treatment of the equine sarcoid. In Practice 1995;17:123–129.

27. French DA, Fretz PB, Davis GD. Mandibular adamantinoma in a horse: radical surgical treatment. Vet Surg 1984;13:165–171.

28. Turrel JM. Oncology. In: Kobluk CN, Ames TR, Geor RJ, eds. The Horse: Diseases and Clinical Management. Philadelphia: WB Saunders, 1995:1128–1130.

29. Orsini JA, Nunamaker DM, Jones CJ, Acland HM. Excision of an oral squamous carcinoma in a horse. Vet Surg 1991;20:264–266.

30. Paterson S. Treatment of superficial ulcerative squamous cell carcinoma in three horses with topical 5-fluorouracil. Vet Rec 1997;141:6626–6628.

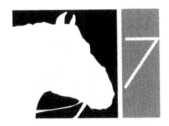

GERIATRIC HORSE DENTISTRY

KRISTIN WILEWSKI, TONY BASILE, AND PATRICIA PENCE

Geriatric horses are horses that are 20 years old or older. Equine practitioners are seeing more geriatric patients now than in the past for several reasons: Horses are not used for transportation and long days of excruciating hard work, so they are not physically worn out and crippled at a young age, as they used to be. Another reason is that equine healthcare is more sophisticated. Parasite control, vaccination against infectious disease, the development of antibiotics, and anti-inflammatory medication have also contributed to prolonging and improving the quality of life of horses. Older horses that are gentle and well-trained are considered to have value as mounts for children, inexperienced riders, the handicapped, and people with poor balance and fragile bones like the elderly. Finally, horse owners in our times are likely to be people who are more affluent and who regard horses as pets or even family members. They are more sentimentally attached to their horses and less likely to send a healthy old saddle gelding or barren brood mare to slaughter.

Geriatric horses have special dental problems related to the constant attrition of reserve crown. In addition, horses that have experienced a lifetime of dental neglect, combined with orthodontic abnormalities, can have severe pathology in the form of abnormal tooth structure and periodontal disease. The goal of this chapter is to introduce the practitioner to situations commonly encountered when performing dentistry on older horses.

PREDENTAL EXAMINATION

Before performing any dental work, the practitioner should have a discussion with the client about possible complications, postdentistry care, and special diets that may be needed. A complete physical examination should be performed, and a CBC and chemistry profile is highly recommended even in apparently healthy horses. Preexisting cardiac, pulmonary, renal, and hepatic disease should be revealed so appropriate decisions can be made regarding sedation and prognosis of postdentistry recovery. The horse's legs should be examined to see if the horse can lock the legs in extension and remain standing during sedation. Severely arthritic joints, especially carpal joints, may not be able to completely extend and lock.

A comprehensive health examination is especially important in horses that are thin and debilitated. Their physical condition may be so marginal that instead of putting on weight, they may decline rapidly after the stress of extensive dentistry. If they are not already on a special diet that is nutritionally complete and requires little mastication, they should be put on one for several weeks before extensive dental procedures. This not only gives them a chance to build up some reserves, but will also determine whether they will even eat the new diet. Some old horses can be very stubborn about eating new food. It would not be kind to either the horse or the owner to perform dentistry on a thin, unhealthy old horse that could not reap its benefits.

KEY POINT:
▶ Make any necessary dietary changes before extensive dental procedures to ensure that the horse will eat the new food.

■ ■ **DIET**

As with horses of any age, geriatric horses need a diet that is nutritionally complete and formulated for their specific needs. They also need roughage. If the horse cannot masticate long-stemmed baled hay into small enough particles to prevent impaction, then the horse must be fed differently. Several major manufacturers of equine concentrated feeds offer pellet diets that are formulated for the older horse *(Box 7.1)*. If the horse has no functional teeth, or no teeth at all, select a diet that can be mixed with water to make a mush.

BOX 7.1 FEEDS AND CALORIE SUPPLEMENTS FOR SENIOR HORSES		
Purina Equine Senior	Alfalfa cubes (not pellets)	Beet pulp (soaked)
Equine Advantage	Rice bran	Corn or canola oil
Nutrena Senior		

Roughage can be fed as hay cubes (not hay pellets) that are soaked in water if necessary. Horses need a certain amount of roughage in their diets to feel "full." Rice bran is a good source of additional fiber and fat.

It is important that the owner understand how much of the pellet food they will have to feed. If the diet consists completely of a senior feed, then the horse may have to eat as much as 18 to 20 lbs. a day, which is nearly half a bag of feed in some cases. The feed should be put into a container and weighed so the owner will see how much needs to be fed at each feeding. All too often the senior horse loses weight when it is put on one of these diets because the owner has no concept of how much pellet food it takes to maintain or gain weight.

■■ SEDATION, RESTRAINT, AND SUPPORT

When working on older horses, you need to consider their temperament and response to sedation. Some of these senior horses that are normally docile and obedient become stubborn and resentful of your interference with their daily routine. Once sedated, these horses exhibit odd avoidance behaviors in which they resist you by leaning back on their hocks, dropping the front end in a "bowing" posture, or by curving their torsos into impossible positions. Sometimes they will even lie down to prevent being worked on.

If possible, use a set of stocks when performing dentistry on geriatric horses. Use long, soft, cotton ropes or nylon webbing to create a sling under the belly, and have stock doors, chains, or ropes on the front and back ends of the stocks. Then the horse can lean back or even sit on the back of the stocks. Belly ropes remove the option of lying down. Once they realize they can't avoid the procedure, most geriatric horses give up and stand fairly well.

PRACTICE TIP
When sedating a horse that is older than 25 years, keep in mind that it may metabolize the drugs slower and that it may become unsteady on its feet. Start with 25% less sedative (by volume) than you would for a younger horse of equivalent weight. Wait a full 5 minutes before stimulating the horse in any way. If you have to give the remaining 25% to get the desired effect, wait another 5 minutes before starting to work.

You may need to reverse the sedative for several reasons: 1. The horse is too deeply sedated and continuously tries to lie down. 2. The horse is taking too long to recover and has to be taken home. 3. The owner doesn't feel comfortable letting you leave the facility before the horse is more awake. 4. The horse develops a severe arrhythmia or other cardiovascular condition that requires reversal of the sedative.

Yohimbine or tolazoline can be given with caution to reverse the sedative. Give yohimbine (0.1 mg/kg) or tolazoline (4.0 mg/kg) slowly over a full minute or longer.[1]

■ ■ MALOCCLUSIONS

Geriatric horses can have the same dental conformation faults and malocclusions that mature horses have, i.e., wave mouth, hooks, ramps, and incisor misalignments. Step mouth, i.e., cheek teeth of uneven length without a common pattern, is more common in geriatric horses. Spaces are created by missing teeth, loose teeth, and abnormally erupted teeth *(Fig. 7.1A–C)*. If these spaces appear when the horse is in its late teens or younger, the opposing teeth will erupt and wear into the gaps *(Fig. 7.2A and B)*. Overlong cheek teeth (hooks, ramps, and waves) can be a centimeter or longer than other teeth in the arcade and can cause gingival or even bone abnormalities in the opposing arcade *(Fig. 7.3A and B)*. Incisors can be severely overgrown, misaligned, or normal. If the horse has been cribbing for most of its life, then the upper incisors may be considerably shorter than the lower incisors.

There are instances in which severe waves in a geriatric horse should not be completely corrected. If the #108–109, 208–209 teeth are severely worn down, it will do no good to completely reduce the #308–309, 408–409, because the upper teeth cannot erupt down to fill the gap. Trying to completely correct these abnormalities in a horse is contraindicated if it will take the teeth completely out of occlusion for the remainder of the horse's life. If the teeth in the wave malocclusion are tight, address the cupped teeth, remove the sharp points, and then check occlusion. If the incisors are not too long, the occlusion may be sufficient for the horse to masticate adequately.

If the teeth are healthy, not severely overgrown, and are still solid in the alveolus, most of the techniques used to correct the teeth of younger horses can be applied to those of the geriatric horse. However, percussion cutters like the Equi-Chip are not recommended in geriatric horses because the abrupt blow required to cut the tooth may loosen it or even knock it out of the alveolus.

■ ■ PERIODONTAL DISEASE

Periodontal disease is common in geriatric horses.[2–6] The primary cause of periodontal disease in the horse is the presence of dental abnormalities that prevent normal occlusion and normal mastication.[6] One examiner found that 60% of horses over the age of 15 years had some degree of periodontal disease.[8] Some periodontal

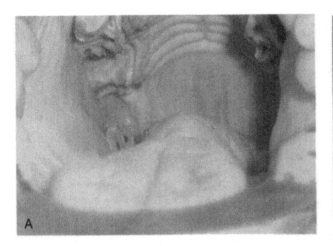

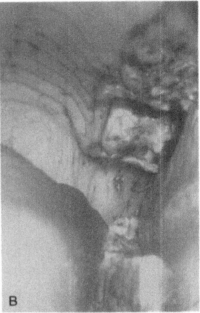

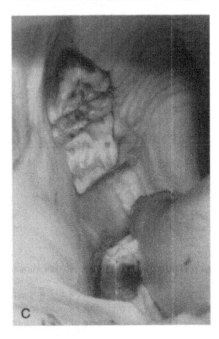

Figure 7.1 Examples of step-mouth abnormalities in three geriatric horses of unknown ages. Color plates **A.** This horse is presumed to be older than 30 years. None of the teeth were functional. The loose teeth were extracted, and those that were not loose had sharp edges removed and overlong areas reduced. Note the extremely overlong tooth in the 4th quadrant. There is a chronic wound in the palate where this tooth lacerated the soft tissue when the horse attempted lateral excursions of the mandible. The overlong tooth had erupted into a gap between two upper teeth. **B.** The distal half of the #208 tooth is missing. The opposing areas of #308 and 309 have erupted into the space. **C.** The distal half of #108 and the medial half of #109 have erupted into a gap in the 4th quadrant. Also notice the unusual saw-tooth pattern of wear in the 6s, 7s, and 8s created by excessive transverse ridges.

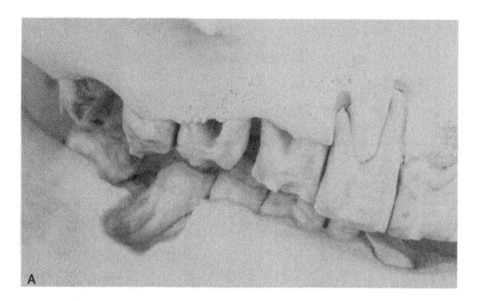

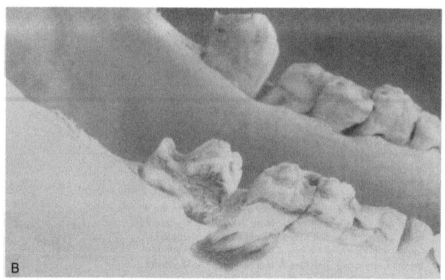

Figure 7.2 Quadrants 1 and 4 in a geriatric horse. The bone overlying #410 has been removed to show the length of the roots. **A.** Teeth #106 and #107 have been dominant over #406 and #407 throughout the life of this horse. The result is that #406 and #407 were prematurely worn to the roots. All remnants of #406 are gone. The only remnant of #407 is a fragment of the distal root. Notice the large gaps between #108–109, #110–111, and #410–411. Note also the bone erosion and porous appearance and erosion of the bone associated with #108 and #109. This could have been caused by severe periodontal disease from food packing in the space between #108–109. **B.** The same horse without the maxilla. Notice the unusual wear pattern on #411 created by overgrowth of the medial aspect into the gap left in the medial part of #111. Notice also how the #309 and #310 teeth in the opposite hemimandibel have drifted into abnormal positions. Tooth #311 is overlong because #211 is absent.

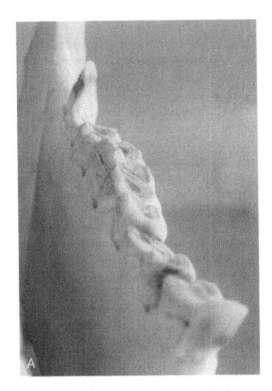

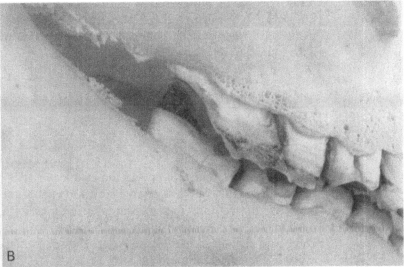

Figure 7.3 Wavey molars and very long hooks on the lower 11s were present in this horse that was about 33 years old. **A.** Lower left arcade. The lower 6s and 7s were worn to the roots. In spite of the overwear of the lower 6s by overlong upper 6s, the medial aspects of the 6s wore into a ramp conformation, which gives them the appearance of being hooks.
B. Lateral view of the upper and lower right arcade of the same horse.

disease may be inevitable because teeth taper from crown to root. By the time the horse enters its geriatric years, the interproximal spaces may have widened and become pockets for food and plaque buildup. See Chapter 10, Dental Infections.

Signs of periodontal disease include halitosis, difficulty eating, gingival hyperemia, edema, and ulceration. Horses with periodontal disease have also been reported to quid hay, but not green grass[2] Dixon Lane. It is not unusual in geriatric horses for periodontal disease to be advanced; the gingival attachments broken at the gingival margin result in formation of food-filled periodontal pockets. Subgingival plaque and calculus deposits build up on the exposed reserve crown and cause the irritation, edema, and ulceration to extend apically and erode the alveolar bone *(Figs. 7.2A and 7.3B)*.[6]

Treatment of periodontal disease in the geriatric horse involves correcting the occlusal abnormalities as much as possible, extracting extremely loose and split teeth, removing tartar, and debriding the periodontal pockets. Packing the pockets with antibiotic gel is a treatment modality that is currently being evaluated.

■ ■ BENIGN GINGIVAL HYPERPLASIA

These are tumor-like masses that develop from the fibrous tissue of the gingival mucosa.[6] They are usually caused by chronic tissue irritation from infection or tartar. They can also be caused by severely overlong teeth irritating the opposing mucosal tissue. See Case Report #4. They can be removed surgically and usually don't recur if the causative factors are eliminated.

■ ■ CHEEK TEETH

Loose Cheek Teeth

Invariably, cheek teeth will appear looser in a geriatric horse than they will in a younger horse. There is less reserve crown to anchor the teeth within the alveoli. Moreover, the teeth are tapered toward the root apex. As the teeth become narrower, small gaps appear between them that impinge upon the integrity of the arcade. These gaps allow food particles to collect and set the stage for periodontal disease, which further attacks the anchor.

Loose cheek teeth should be identified during the dental examination. Loose cheek teeth will make a *squeaking* sound when lateral excursion is checked by manipulating the mandible. After the full-mouth speculum is put into place, each cheek tooth should be grasped with the fingers and wiggled. Another way to detect loose cheek teeth is to gently run a float over the arcade. Loose teeth will sound *hollow* compared with well-anchored teeth.

Just because a tooth is loose does not mean it must be extracted. It is the opinion of the authors that some teeth will tighten up if they are unloaded, i.e., taken slightly out of occlusion by reducing the occlusal surface.

Which teeth should the practitioner extract, and which teeth should be unloaded and given a chance to tighten up? Although there are no studies to verify these criteria, anecdotal reports suggest a rule of thumb: If the tooth can be wiggled with the fingers, try applying a wiggling pressure to the occlusal surface using a large dental probe. If it can be wiggled with the dental probe, it is too loose and should be extracted. If it cannot be wiggled using the probe, unload the tooth and leave it. Clean out periodontal pockets and treat periodontal disease as described in Chapter 10, Dental Infections.

KEY POINT:
▶ Unloading a loose tooth by taking it slightly out of occlusion may extend the functional life of the tooth.

PRACTICE TIP
Loose teeth make a *squeaking* sound when lateral mandibular excursion is checked and a *hollow* sound when a float is rasped over them.

Extracting loose teeth is usually a simple procedure in the geriatric horse, because there is so little reserve crown remaining to anchor the tooth. Molar spreaders are rarely needed, and extremely loose teeth can be removed with cap extractors. If there are still strong gingival attachments, use a dental pick to elevate the gingiva. Broad-spectrum antibiotics should be considered in all horses that have teeth extracted. If during the predental physical examination a heart murmur is detected, antibiotics should be started at least 1 day before the procedure.

Once the tooth has been extracted, the opposing tooth must be reduced to level with the arcade and dental exams should be scheduled every 6 months to prevent the opposing tooth from overerupting into the space left by the extracted tooth. Teeth usually erupt more slowly in the geriatric mouth and there may be little change between visits, but occasionally sudden changes do occur, especially if the overall health of the horse is declining.

PRACTICE TIP
Molar cutters make useful extractors in animals with small oral cavities when a low-profile instrument is needed. It doesn't take as much force to grasp a tooth as it takes to cut through one.

Multiple Loose Cheek Teeth

If there are a lot of loose cheek teeth that need to be removed, the condition and usefulness of the remaining tight teeth need to be assessed. If there are three or more adjacent tight teeth that are opposed by three or more adjacent tight teeth on the opposing arcade, these teeth should be balanced and floated as well as possible and left in place.

If, however, the remaining tight teeth do not form a useful battery of teeth, a decision must be made about whether to extract them, or cut or burr them shorter and leave them in place. At the present time, there is no agreement regarding whether nonfunctional teeth that are still tight should be left in place or removed. Some practitioners believe that it is too traumatic to a geriatric horse to perform multiple extractions of teeth that are still well-seated, whereas others believe it is a relief to the horse to not have a few useless cheek teeth left in its mouth, especially if they are associated with severe gingivitis.

The *clean-out* procedure involves extracting the remaining maxillary cheek teeth and cutting or burring the remaining mandibular teeth to nearly gum level. See Case Report #2. The alveoli of maxillary teeth heal faster and with fewer complications after extraction than do mandibular teeth because gravity allows them to drain freely. Cutting or burring down the mandibular teeth rather than extracting them gets them out of the way and reduces healing time. A less traumatic compromise would be to cut or burr all the remaining teeth short enough that they do not cause trauma to the gingiva of the opposing arcade. It is imperative to already have the horse eating a complete pelleted diet and alfalfa cubes before any traumatic procedure is performed.

As always, after the cheek teeth are worked on, the incisors are realigned and balanced. In this case, however, they would not be cut any shorter.

Cupped Cheek Teeth

Most horses over the age of 25 years will have teeth that are expired, i.e., worn down to the bottom of the reserve crown and no longer erupting. These teeth are usually still held tightly in the alveoli; have a smooth, enamel-free appearance to the center of the tooth; and have a rim on the lingual, mesial, distal, and buccal edges. Often more than one tooth is involved, and sometimes the entire arcade can have this appearance *(Fig. 7.4)*. These teeth will never again be fully functional but may still be useful to the horse. The ridges must be reduced because they interfere with lateral excursion. Do not reduce them to the level of the center of the tooth, which is usually too short compared with the rest of the arcade. The opposing teeth are usually too long and may need to be reduced. Restore the table angles after reducing the rims.

Split and Broken Cheek Teeth

Teeth that are split or broken into the pulp should be extracted *(Fig. 7.5)*. The gingival attachments may still be secure and may need to be elevated with a dental probe. Root fragment extractors may be needed to remove all the pieces if the tooth fragments during extraction. After extraction, flush the socket with dilute antiseptic and administer antibiotics.

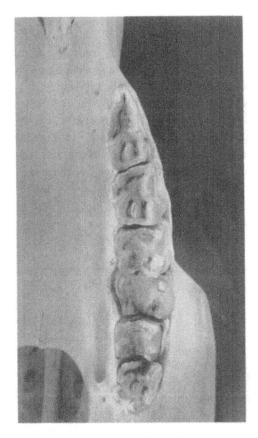

Figure 7.4 Occlusal view of the upper left arcade in a geriatric horse. Although difficult to appreciate in a photograph, all of the teeth have cupped occlusal surfaces and sharp enamel rims in the outer enamel. Teeth #208 to 210 are wearing into the roots, as can be seen by the lack of enamel and infundibular structures in the center of the occlusal surfaces.

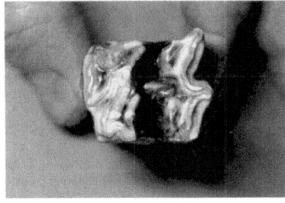

Figure 7.5 Photo of split maxillary tooth. (Reprinted with permission from Knottenbelt, Colour Atlas of Diseases and Disorders of the Horse. St. Louis: Mosby, 1994.)

Geriatric horses can have the same incisor misalignments seen in younger horses, i.e., dorsal curvature, ventral curvature, slant, overbite, underbite, and step mouth *(Figs. 7.6 and 7.7)* The incisors should be realigned and rebalanced if needed. It is important to not overreduce the incisors in geriatric horses because they are more likely to have compromised cheek teeth. Full molar contact and pressure on compromised teeth can be uncomfortable and eventually loosen the teeth. It is considered acceptable to leave the older horse with slightly more incisor length and correspondingly less molar occlusion than you would leave in younger horses. Geriatric horses tend to need incisor realignment less frequently than younger horses.

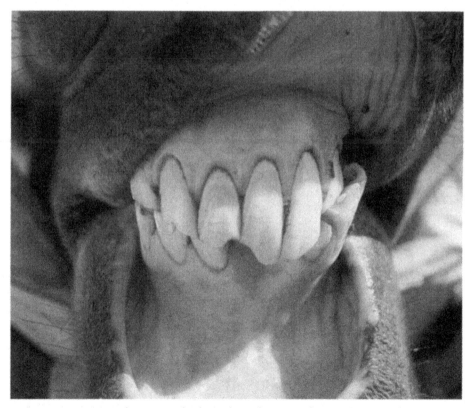

Figure 7.6 Incisor misalignments. This horse has a large gap between #301 and 401 created by an old injury, a split mandibular symphysis. Although it appears at first glance that there are several lower incisors missing, they are all there. Teeth #101 and 102 have erupted into what may have originally been a much smaller space and have widened the gap.

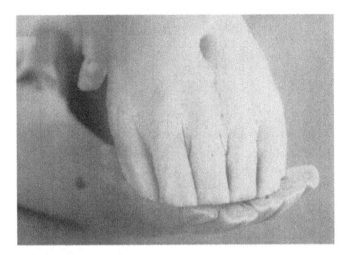

Figure 7.7 This is the same horse as in Figure 7.3. The horse had a slant bite in its youth. As the angle of eruption of the incisors became steeper in its geriatric years, the slant bite wore into more of a wry bite conformation.

KEY POINT:
▶ Do not overreduce incisors in geriatric horses. This puts too much stress on the cheek teeth and may loosen them.

Loose Incisors

Unlike the cheek teeth, loose incisors are not usually a problem in geriatric horses. If loose incisors are discovered, then they should be extracted and the opposing teeth reduced to level or slightly shorter than level with the adjacent incisors. In rare cases in which all the incisors are loose, they can all be extracted, but it is the author's experience that horses appear to have a harder time adjusting to having no incisors than they do to having no cheek teeth (Wilewski). This may be due to the increased pressure on the cheek teeth and the temporomandibular joint.

■ ■ **ARTHRITIS OF THE TEMPOROMANDIBULAR JOINT**

Arthritic changes of the temporomandibular joint (TMJ) can be seen in horse skulls. The changes range from periarticular lipping at the bone-joint capsule interface to severe malformations of the mandibular condyle and opposing articular surface *(Figs. 7.8A and B)*. The most severe abnormalities were associated with shear mouth conditions and fractured mandibles. More work needs to be done to catalog dental abnormalities that result in temporomandibular joint osteoarthritis in order to establish etiologies.

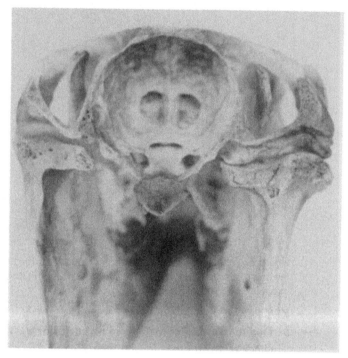

Figure 7.8   Arthritis of the temporomandibular joint.

■ ■ · TUMORS

Neoplasia of the teeth and oral cavity are relatively uncommon in horses. Typically, younger horses are more prone to oral and dental tumors than older horses.[7]

Squamous cell carcinomas are the most common oral neoplasm in the horse. Nonpigmented skin, especially at the mucocutaneous junction of the lips, that is chronically exposed to high levels of ultraviolet light (strong sunlight) is most frequently involved. Clydesdales, Appaloosas, and other breeds with nonpigmented skin of the face and lips are more frequently affected than other breeds. Tumors can also arise in irritated alveolar epithelium in cases of chronic periodontitis.[7,8]

Although these tumors are relatively slow-growing, they are highly invasive and destructive to surrounding structures.[9] It is not unusual for oral squamous cell carcinomas to invade the hard palate, the nasal cavity, and the paranasal sinuses, resulting in altered airflow and gross facial distortion.[8–11]

Diagnosis is by biopsy. Radiography is necessary to identify masses in the sinuses and to help quantify the extent of bone destruction. Treatment modalities involving surgical excision, gamma radiation, and chemotherapy have been described.[12–14]

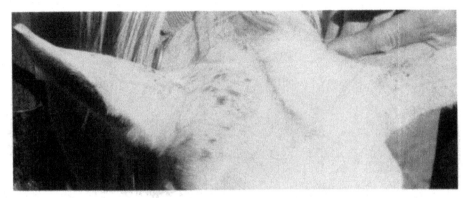

Figure 7.9 Melanoma. This grey horse had asymmetry of the tissues in the temporal region, which could be mistaken for muscle hypertrophy caused by dental abnormalities. It also had melanomas in the commissures of the lips.

Melanomas are tumors of the melanin-producing cells. They are common in gray-colored horses of all ages. Melanomas in gray horses are usually benign and slow growing; however, they can become malignant in old horses. Melanomas of the head region are found on or around the ears, the eyelids, the commissures of the lips, and in the parotid salivary glands *(Fig. 7.9)*. Diagnosis is by clinical presentation and biopsy. Treatment has been described and includes surgical excision, cryonecrosis, biologic response modifiers (cimetidine), and chemotherapy.[15,16]

Case Report #1 *(Figs. 7.10A–G)*

This is a 26-year-old Arab gelding used as a school horse. He has a severe wave mouth due to years of inadequate dentistry. Teeth #106, 206, 310, 311, 410, and 411 were extremely overlong, and the teeth opposing them in the opposite arcade are worn to the gumline or missing. These long teeth were reduced by cutting them down with molar cutters, then burring them level. The decision to use molar cutters was based on the fact that the opposing teeth were either absent or expired and would never be useful to this horse again, therefore it would be no loss if they were loosened by the molar cutters. The #308 and 408 teeth were also overlong, but less severely than the others, and #108 and 208 were correspondingly shortened. These teeth were burred level. The #106 and 206 teeth were also extremely overlong, but it was difficult to cut these teeth with molar cutters. They were reduced to a desirable length using burrs. Because this horse was still being used as a riding horse, bit seats were also created.

In the postdentistry photos, it is still apparent that the teeth are not all level, and the wave mouth is still evident. This is because further reduction would have taken the cheek teeth completely out of occlusion. The shortest teeth in the arcade are in

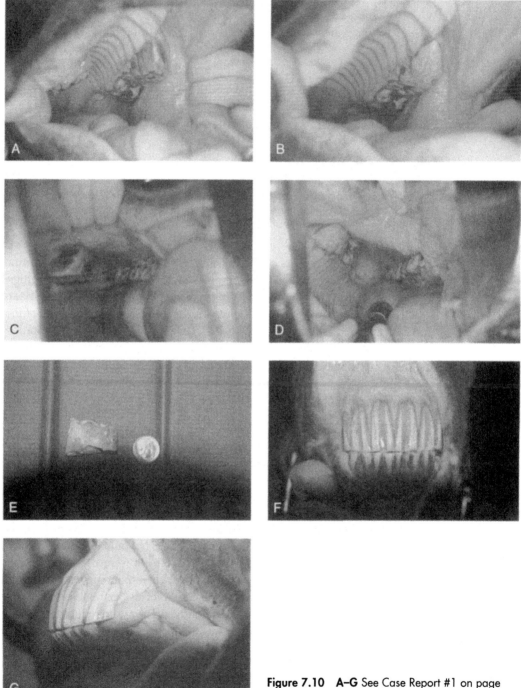

Figure 7.10 A–G See Case Report #1 on page 183 for explanation.

fact too short, so it was not desirable to reduce all the teeth until they were level with each other but too short to be in occlusion. Because of his advanced age and the lack of reserve crown in the remaining cheek teeth, this horse will never have normal molar arcades.

Surprisingly, this horse had relatively normal incisors and only required a minor incisor bite realignment to bring him into good molar occlusion. He had only a small remnant of the #303 tooth left, which was probably an abnormal tooth that had never fully developed. Over the years, the remaining lower incisors had shifted to center themselves, allowing him relatively normal incisor occlusion.

Case Report #2 *(Figs. 7.11A–C)*

This is a 25-year-old quarter horse brood mare. This mare was approximately 150 lbs. over-weight, so the owners did not suspect that she had any dental problems. She had long, beak-like upper #6s. The #206 was so long that it extended to the gingiva of the interdental space of the opposing mandible. There is a rough-surfaced nodule of heperplastic tissue approximately 2 cm in diameter at the site of irritation. The overlong portion of the tooth was cut with a B-head, simple-action molar cutter and the cut surface was smoothed with a ½-inch round carbide burr. This mare also had sharp enamel points on the buccal edges of the upper cheek teeth. The buccal mucosa was thickened and discolored by years of irritation. The hyperplastic tissue was excised after the dental work was performed. There was minimal bleeding at the excision site.

Case Report #3 *(Figs. 7.12A–E)*

This is a 26-year-old retired Appaloosa mare. She had halitosis and ulcerations in her mouth due to multiple loose, split, and cupped teeth. However, she did have some teeth that could form a useful battery. The right side of her mouth was the worst. The #106 and 108 were loose, and the #107 was split and loose. These teeth were easily extracted with cap extractors. The #206, 306, and 406 were also loose and easily extracted. The upper left side had multiple cupped cheek teeth that were still tight. These tight teeth were burred until the lingual and buccal rims did not interfere with lateral excursion. The overlong #111, 211, 307, 308, 309, 407, 408, and 409 were burred until level with the arcades, and the table angles were reestablished. Finally, the remaining teeth were floated and the incisors were realigned.

This mare will never have ideal occlusion again due to the multiple absent cheek teeth, but after this dental, she did have some occlusion on the right side and fairly good occlusion on the left side. Antibiotics and anti-inflammatory medication were prescribed after this dental procedure.

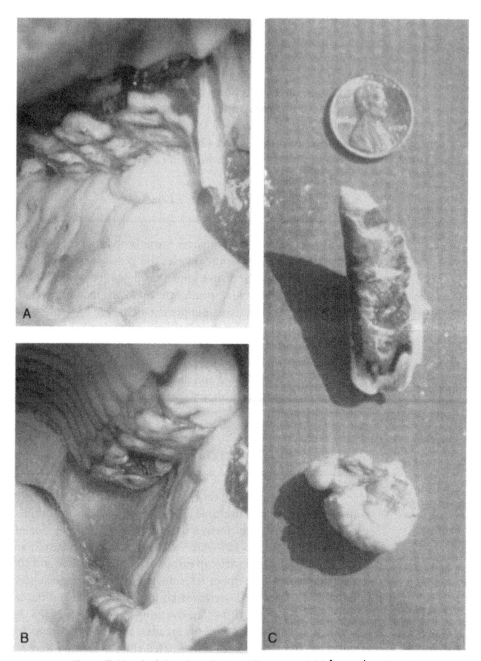

Figure 7.11   A–C See Case Report #2 on page 185 for explanation.

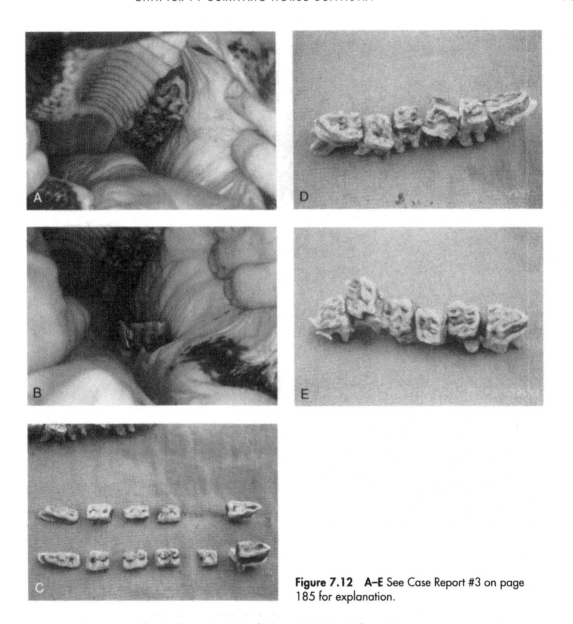

Figure 7.12 **A–E** See Case Report #3 on page 185 for explanation.

Case Report #4 *(Figs. 7.13A–F)*

This is a 37-year-old retired paint mare that was already on a pelleted diet for senior horses. The dental abnormalities were more dramatic on palpation than on visual examination. All the upper cheek teeth were loose. The #107 and #208 were so loose they were extracted with fingers during the palpation examination. The #307

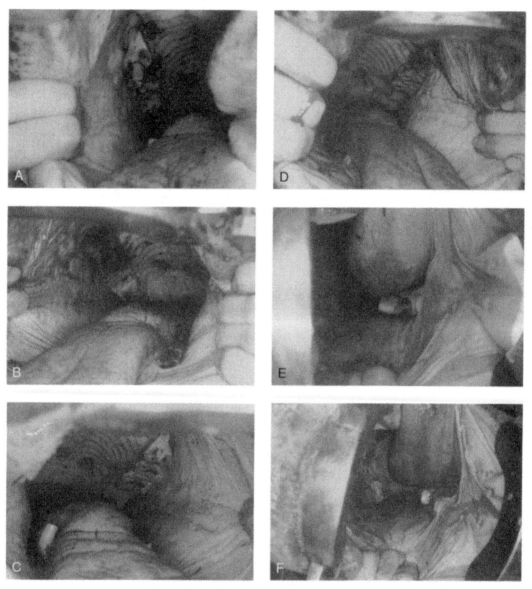

Figure 7.13   A–F See Case Report #4 on page 187 for explanation.

was absent, and the #306 and 406 were also loose. With so many cheek teeth loose, the decision was made to extract all the remaining upper cheek teeth and the #306 and 406. All the remaining lower cheek teeth were cut to the gumline.

This mare also had a slant bite. The incisors were realigned until level to equalize the pressure on the TMJ. The mare was put on antibiotics for 10 days and anti-inflammatory medication as needed.

■■ REFERENCES

1. Gross ME, Tranquilli WJ. Use of alpha 2-adrenergic receptor antagonists. J Am Vet Med Assoc 1989;195:378.
2. Colyer JF. A note on dental diseases in horses. Vet Rec 1905; Sep 23.
3. Little WL. Periodontal disease in the horse. J Comp Pathol 1913;26:240–249.
4. Kirkland KD, Marretta SM, Indue OJ, et al. Survey of equine dental disease and associated oral pathology. In: Proceedings of the 40th Annual Convention of the American Association of Equine Practitioners, Vancouver, 1994.
5. Dixon PM. Equine cheek teeth disease: is periodontal disease still a problem? B Vet Dent Assoc J 1992;2:1–4.
6. Dixon PM. Dental disease. In: Robinson NE, ed. Current Therapy in Equine Medicine. 4th ed. Philadelphia: WB Saunders, 1997.
7. Baker GJ. Abnormalities of wear and periodontal disease. In: Baker GJ, Easley J, eds. Equine dentistry. Philadelphia: WB Saunders, 1999.
8. Baker GJ. Some aspects of equine dental disease. Equine Vet J 1990;2(3):105–110.
9. Knottenbelt DC. Oral and dental tumors. In: Baker GJ, Easley J, eds. Equine Dentistry. Philadelphia: WB Saunders, 1999:85–103.
10. Strafuss AC. Squamous cell carcinoma in horses. J Am Vet Med Assoc 1976;168:61–62.
11. Howie F, Munroe G, Thompson H, Murphy D. Palatine squamous cell carcinoma involving the maxillary sinus in two horses. Equine Vet Ed 1992;4:3–7.
12. Jubb KVF, Kennedy PC, Palmer N. Pathology of Domestic Animals. 4th Ed. New York: Academic Press, 1992:27.
13. Leyland A, Baker JR. Lesions of the nasal cavity and paranasal sinuses of the horse causing dyspnoea. British Vet J 1975;131:339–346.
14. Orsini JA, Nunamaker DM, Jones CJ, Acland HM. Excision of oral squamous cell carcinoma in a horse. Vet Surg 1991;20:264–266.
15. Paterson S. Treatment of superficial ulcerative squamous cell carcinoma in three horses with topical 5-fluorouracil. Vet Rec 1997;141:626–628.
16. Goetz TE, Ogilvie GK, Keegan KG, Johnson PJ. Cimetidine for the treatment of melanoma in three horses. J Am Vet Med Assoc 1990;196:449–452.
17. Goetz TE, Long MT. Treatment of melanoma in horses. Compend of Contin Educ Pract Vet 1993;15:608–610.
18. Theon AP, Pascoe JR, Carlson GP, et al. Intratumoral chemotherapy with cisplatin in oil emulsion in horses. J Am Vet Med Assoc 1993;202:261–267.

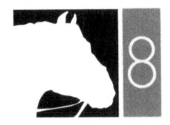

MINIATURE HORSE DENTISTRY

PATRICIA PENCE AND CARL MITZ

Miniature horses present special challenges for the equine dentist. Few owners or practitioners have working facilities for miniatures, so procedures are often performed on hands and knees *(Fig. 8.1)*. Miniatures can be unruly if not taught to be submissive and may require sedation to prevent injury to themselves or their handlers. Abnormalities such as severe crowding of teeth *(Fig. 8.2)*, impactions, and congenital defects are not unusual *(Figs. 8.3, 8.4)*. These abnormalities make frequent examinations and corrective procedures necessary. Finally, their oral cavities are tiny in comparison to a full-sized horse or pony, making it difficult to get instruments and hands inside the mouth to do the dental work. Performing dentistry on the smallest minis has been compared to building a ship in a bottle.

KEY POINT:
▶ Overcrowded teeth, impactions, maleruptions, and congenital defects are the major issues in miniature horse dentistry.

■■ COMMON DENTAL ABNORMALITIES IN MINIATURE HORSES

Although the heads and bodies of miniature horses are scaled-down versions of full-sized horses, the teeth of many of them are not. The teeth can be too large for the smaller, shorter skulls and tiny muzzles. This overcrowding makes delayed eruption and impactions common and difficult to resolve in miniatures.

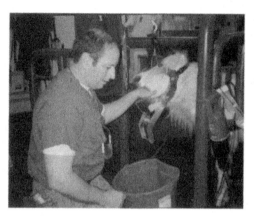

Figure 8.1   Dental procedures on miniature horses are often performed on hands and knees due to lack of specialized work areas. (Photograph courtesy of Tony Basile.)

Signs of impaction include a puffy appearance on one or both sides of the bridge of the nose caused by pronounced eruption cysts *(Fig. 8.5)*, swellings on the ventral mandible, unilateral or sometimes bilateral nasal discharge, foul breath, difficulty eating, and weight loss. It is not unusual to see sinusitis secondary to impacted upper cheek teeth in horses up to 6 and 7 years old. Radiographs may show

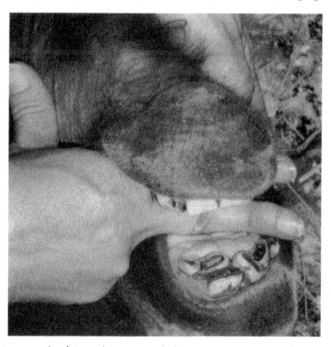

Figure 8.2   An example of severely overcrowded incisors in a miniature horse. (Photograph courtesy of Carl Mitz.)

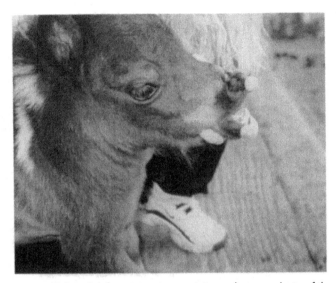

Figure 8.3 Congenital dental defects in a young miniature horse: aplasia of the upper incisors. (Photograph courtesy of Carl Mitz.)

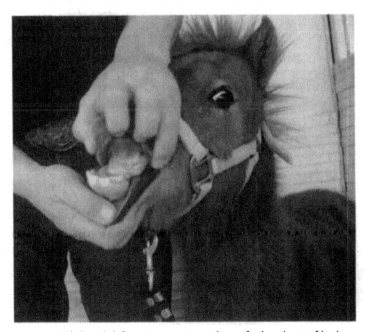

Figure 8.4 Congenital dental defects in a miniature horse foal: aplasia of both upper and lower incisors. (Photograph courtesy of Carl Mitz.)

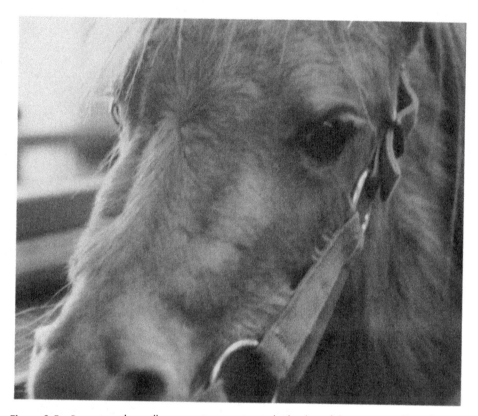

Figure 8.5 Pronounced maxillary eruption cysts give the bridge of the nose a puffy or lumpy appearance. The most common causes are overcrowding of molars and delayed shedding of deciduous molars. (Photograph courtesy of Carl Mitz.)

widened periapical spaces and loss of detail in periapical tissues if infection is present.

Impaction can cause teeth to erupt in abnormal positions. For example, the fourth permanent upper cheek teeth (#108, #208) may erupt lingually or twisted sideways *(Fig. 8.6)* as they try to find a path between the previously erupted adjacent teeth. Permanent incisors sometimes erupt stacked on top of one another or stick straight out into the mucosa *(Figs. 8.7, 8.8, 8.9)*. Some miniature horses are actually dwarf horses and have congenital defects common to animals with dwarf genes, including mandibular prognathism, or *sow-mouth* deformities *(Fig. 8.10)*.

There is no reliable schedule for the eruption of permanent teeth in miniature horses and it is not unusual to have teeth erupt out of sequence or not at all. Some horses never develop corner incisors *(Fig. 8.11)*. These variations make the normal landmarks for aging by dentition all but useless in miniatures.

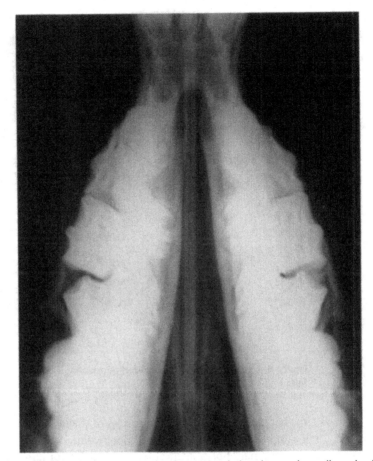

Figure 8.6 Radiographic appearance of overcrowded and twisted maxillary cheek teeth.

KEY POINT:
▶ Abnormal incisor numbers and variable eruption times of cheek teeth can make accurate aging of the miniature horse difficult.

■ ■ DENTAL PROCEDURES

The ideal working situation for routine procedures is to have the miniature horse on an elevated surface high enough for the practitioner to work in a normal seated position. Working for long periods of time on hands and knees is tiring and can strain

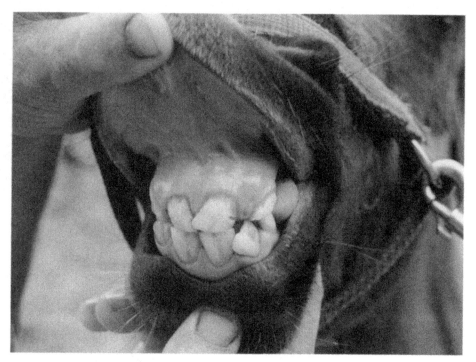

Figure 8.7 Overcrowded and twisted permanent incisors. (Photograph courtesy of Carl Mitz.)

the back, shoulder, and neck muscles of the practitioner. An inexpensive stand with a ramp and stock rails made of pipe, wood, or rope can be made for work done in the veterinary hospital and is recommended for large farms.

Miniature horses require the same prophylactic procedures as full-sized horses, such as floating points and removing deciduous teeth. They also need to have the same corrective procedures performed, including having hooks removed, incisors cut, long teeth reduced, and wavy molars corrected. The main difference in dental care for miniatures concerns removal of deciduous teeth and crowded teeth.

Frequent rechecks should be scheduled for horses due to shed deciduous teeth so they can be removed as early as possible. Timely removal of deciduous teeth may reduce the incidence of impactions, especially in cheek teeth. For horses in which severe overcrowding of permanent incisors or cheek teeth is creating health problems, removal of the offending teeth may be the only solution. The owner should be advised that complications such as infection and incomplete removal of dental material are common following tooth extraction in horses.

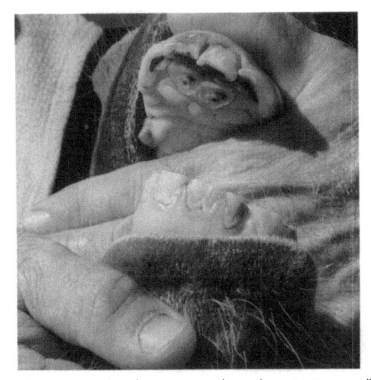

Figure 8.8   Severe overcrowding of incisors can result in teeth erupting in two parallel rows. (Photograph courtesy of Carl Mitz.)

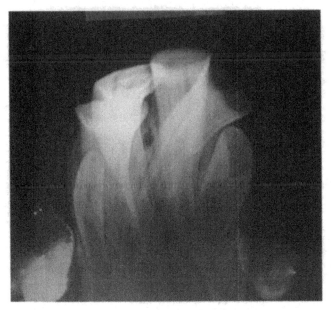

Figure 8.9   Radiographic appearance of overcrowded incisors in a miniature horse.

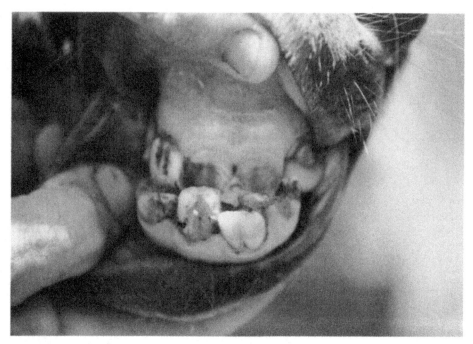

Figure 8.10   Mandibular prognathism in a miniature horse. (Photograph courtesy of Carl Mitz.)

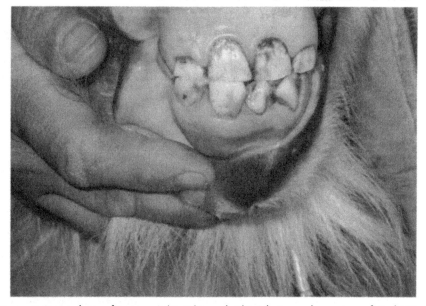

Figure 8.11   Aplasia of incisors 1/3, 2/3, and 4/3. (Photograph courtesy of Carl Mitz.)

■ ■ EQUIPMENT

Several manufacturers make special dental instruments small enough for miniatures. These instruments have low profiles and smaller working surfaces and are more suited for working in the cramped oral cavity. Harlan and World Wide Equine make full-mouth specula for miniatures (see appendix for instrument manufacturers). For practitioners that only occasionally work on miniatures, routine dental procedures, i.e., floating points, reducing long teeth, and cutting incisors can usually be done with the same instruments made for full-sized horses. Even the full-mouth speculum can be used in miniatures, after a few extra holes are made in the straps. When using full-sized instruments, however, extra care should be taken to avoid soft-tissue damage. Use shorter strokes with hand tools, and stop to check your work often when using power instruments. The exceptions are the tiniest minis or those with very refined heads. It is difficult to get anything but the smallest, flattest file in the buccal space of their mouths.

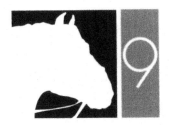

BASICS OF DIAGNOSTIC IMAGING

PATRICIA PENCE

Identifying structures within the equine head that are involved in pathology is an important part of clinical evaluation and is often a challenge. The teeth involved can be difficult to identify even in the presence of swelling and draining tracts primarily because the location of reserve crowns vary with the age of the horse.[1,2] The severity of the pathology and the involvement of adjacent structures frequently cannot be determined by palpation or direct visualization.

Various imaging modalities can be used to isolate the structures of interest, including radiography, computed tomography, nuclear scintigraphy, and ultrasonography. The choice of imaging technology depends on availability and convenience of equipment; whether soft tissue, mineralized tissue, or both need to be examined; and finally whether the cost of diagnosis is justified by the information received. See *Figures 9.1 to 9.5* for examples of dental and associated pathology identified using different imaging modalities.

The purpose of this chapter is to provide tips for taking successful radiographs of the head. Comprehensive radiographic studies and their interpretation have been published by other authors.[3–10] The dental practitioner is encouraged to obtain for reference a collection of radiographic studies of both normal and abnormal structures of the head.

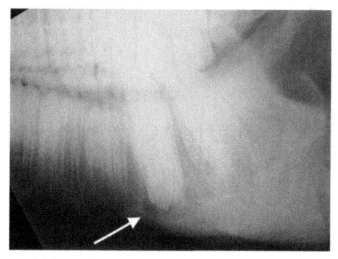

Figure 9.1   Lateral radiographic projection centered over the 1st molar of the lower mandible. There is periapical osteolysis surrounded by a zone of sclerosis and destruction of the tooth root. A radiolucent draining tract can be visualized ventrally (arrow). (Courtesy of Dr. Russ Tucker.)

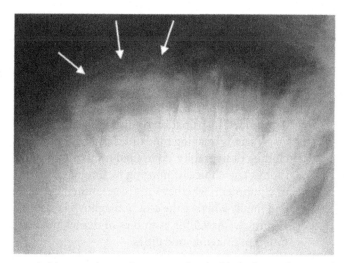

Figure 9.2   Lateral oblique radiograph positioned to highlight the tooth roots of the upper right arcade. There is destruction of the root of the 4th premolar with an expansive ossifying mass (arrows). (Courtesy of Dr. Russ Tucker.)

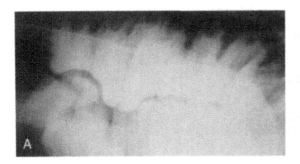

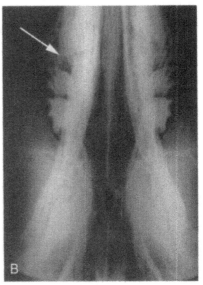

Figure 9.3 A. Lateral radiographic view centered over the occlusal surfaces of the cheek teeth. There is malposition of the lower 2nd premolar teeth with irregular wear of several occlusal surfaces. **B.** Dorsal ventral radiographic projection of the same horse. The abnormal position and wear is evident (arrow). (Courtesy of Dr. Russ Tucker.)

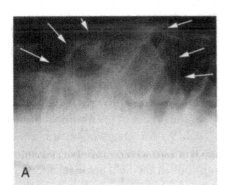

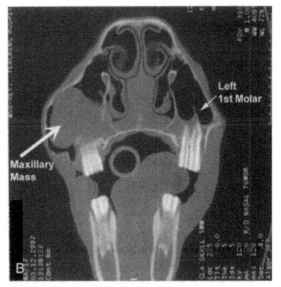

Figure 9.4 A. Lateral oblique radiograph centered over the 1st molar tooth root. There is an expansive mass destroying the tooth root and creating an increased opacification within the maxillary sinus (arrows). **B.** Computed tomographic transverse image of the horse in Figure A at the level of the upper 1st molar teeth. A large soft-tissue mass occupies the right maxillary sinus. The entire tooth root of the 1st molar has been destroyed. Note the normal appearance of the 1st molar and maxillary sinus on the left side. (Courtesy of Dr. Russ Tucker.)

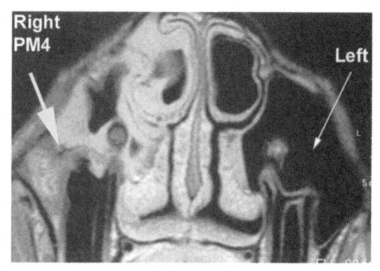

Figure 9.5   Transverse magnetic resonance image (proton density) of a horse at the level of the 4th premolar teeth. There is a large amount of high signal fluid in the right maxillary sinus. Left-sided deviation of the dorsal nasal septum is present. The root of the right 4th premolar has apical erosion. The left side is normal. (Courtesy of Dr. Russ Tucker.)

■ ■ RADIOGRAPHY

Radiography is the primary imaging modality for evaluating osseous structures in veterinary medicine because the equipment is affordable and most practitioners have adequate training in its use. Radiography is ideal for evaluating structures of the head because the various densities of soft tissue, dental tissue, bone, and air can be used to highlight areas of interest by careful positioning of the film or the head of the animal. Multiple oblique views may be necessary to obtain diagnostic films for evaluation of dental structures.

Radiography has its challenges. Due to the long exposure times required by most portable machines, motion blurring is a common problem, originating either from the horse, the holder of the cassette, or the holder of the machine. Multiple exposures and retakes are common. (See *Table 9.1* for suggested techniques and exposure times.) The distance of the patient from the processing area can increase diagnostic time and expenses. Even if conditions in the field are ideal and diagnostic films are obtained, they can be made unreadable by the conditions of the practitioner's darkroom and chemicals. Automatic processors help eliminate processing artifacts. In spite of the disadvantages, radiography remains the most convenient and least expensive imaging method available. When used appropriately, radiography can provide valuable information.

TABLE 9.1   Suggested Technique Chart for Dental Radiography Using a 26-Inch Film-Focal Distance and a 400-Speed Rare-Earth Screen-Film Combination[5]

Projection	Film Type	Time	
		90 kVp, 10 mA 80 kVp, 20 mA	90 kVp, 15 mA
Dorsoventral	PDG *	0.4	0.3
	EM-1#	0.6	0.5
Lateral	PDG	0.2	0.1–0.15
	EM-1	0.3	0.25
Oblique	PDG	0.1–0.15	0.08–0.1
	EM-1	0.2	0.2

*PDG film, Eastman Kodak, Rochester, NY 14650
EM-1 film, Eastman Kodak, Rochester, NY 14650

■■   TECHNIQUE TIPS FOR SUCCESSFUL DENTAL RADIOGRAPHY

1. Have the horse hauled to the facility with the processing equipment when possible.
2. Use a thin rope halter in place of a halter with metal hardware to restrain the horse.
3. Use low kV, high mA technique for increased contrast between soft tissue and osseous structures.
4. Use a 26-inch film-focal distance and a 400-speed or higher rare-earth screen-film combination.[5]
5. Subject motion can be reduced by sedating the horse and supporting its head with a dental headstand. Some horses may require a blindfold as well. General anesthesia may be required in some horses for difficult views.
6. Collimate the x-ray beam as tightly as possible to avoid loss of detail from scattered radiation.
7. Cassette motion can be reduced by supporting the cassette in a cassette holder with a handle, a cassette stand, or by placing the cassette in a bag suspended from an IV stand.[3] This also keeps the assistant holding the cassette out of the direct line of exposure.
8. If the x-ray machine is not mounted on a tube support, motion can be reduced by supporting the x-ray machine on a ladder, trash can, saw horse, or other type of fixed support.[3]

TABLE 9.2   Radiographic Views for Equine Dental Examinations[3-10]

Structures to Examine	View
Incisors, canines, premaxilla, and rostral mandible	Lateral
	Dorsoventral
Premaxilla	Intraoral-dorsoventral
Rostral mandible	Intraoral-ventrodorsal
Horizontal rami-mandible and lower cheek teeth	Lateral
	Ventral 45-degree lateral-dorsolateral oblique
Upper cheek teeth	Dorsal 60-degree lateral-dorsolateral oblique
Nasal cavity and paranasal sinuses	Lateral
	Dorsal 60-degree lateral-dorsolateral oblique
Lateral aspect of maxillary sinus	Dorsoventral
Maxillary sinus	Dorsal 15-degree lateral-ventrolateral oblique
Temporomandibular joint	Lateral

9. Cassettes should be placed on the diseased side of the head to minimize distortion and magnification.
10. Oblique views prevent superimposition of contralateral dental structures. Mentally visualize the desired image of the structures, and adjust the obliqueness of the cassette and machine accordingly. **See *Table 9.2*** for descriptions of radiographic views.
11. Identical views of the contralateral side for comparison can be helpful when the pathology of a structure is in doubt.
12. Contrast radiography can help identify the source of a draining tract. The simplest contrast agent is a metal teat cannula inserted into the tract.[4]

■ ■   RADIOGRAPHIC SIGNS OF DENTAL DISEASE[2,3]

1. Bone lysis, i.e., lysis of lamina dura, lysis around tooth apex, lytic tracts extending from mandibular tooth roots.
2. Bone production, i.e., sclerosis and opacities adjacent to the tooth apex (cementum granulomas).
3. Periosteal reaction.
4. Displacement of normal structures, i.e., displacement of teeth, fracture lines, distortion, or expansion of bone cortices.
5. Abnormal air pockets.
6. Soft-tissue mineralization.
7. Widening of the periodontal membrane.

8. Abnormal shape of tooth root, i.e., *clubbing* of tooth root, or *halo* around tooth root.
9. Air-fluid interfaces in the sinuses.
10. Soft-tissue opacities in sinuses and nasal conchae.

■ ■ COMPUTED TOMOGRAPHY[11,12]

Transverse cross sections of the head can be obtained in 1 to 10 mm slices and can be digitally reconstructed into sagittal, dorsal, or three-dimensional views, enabling the borders of lesions to be precisely identified. Resolution is excellent for osseous and dental details and is good for some soft-tissue structures. Differentiating between neoplastic and necrotic lesions is facilitated by using contrast CT to examine blood perfusion. The major disadvantages to using CT to image dental pathology are that it requires transporting the horse to a university or major equine veterinary referral center, that the horse must be subjected to somewhat lengthy general anesthesia, and that it is expensive.

■ ■ ULTRASONOGRAPHY[13]

Ultrasonography is not well suited for exploring dental lesions, but it can be used to examine soft-tissue swelling in the head. It is especially helpful for guiding needle aspirates and biopsy instruments to investigate swelling in the throat latch and pharyngeal regions.

■ ■ NUCLEAR SCINTIGRAPHY[14]

Nuclear scintigraphy is not commonly used to image lesions in the head. However, it can be useful when pathology is suspected but cannot be confirmed by other imaging modalities. Nuclear scintigraphy is very sensitive, but lacks specificity in lesion detection. Resolution is very poor, so fine osseous details cannot be seen; however, nuclear bone scans are extremely sensitive to changes in bone. Radioisotope-tagged leukocyte scans can be used to locate areas of infections, including abscesses. Obvious disadvantages involve availability of special facilities and licensing, use of radioactive materials, and expense. Following nuclear scintigraphy, horses are typically required to stay in radiation isolation facilities for 24 to 48 hours.

Acknowledgments. Special thanks to Russell Tucker, DVM, ACVR, DIPL for reviewing earlier versions of this chapter.

■ ■ **REFERENCES**

1. Kirkland KD, Baker GJ, Marretta SM, et al. Effects of aging on the endodontic system, reserve crown, and roots of equine mandibular cheek teeth. Am J Vet Res 1996;57:31–38.
2. Dixon PM, Copeland AN. The radiological appearance of mandibular cheek teeth in ponies of different ages. Equine Vet Educ 1993;5:317–323.
3. Gibbs C. Dental imaging. In: Baker GJ, Easley J, eds. Equine dentistry. Philadelphia: WB Saunders, 1999.
4. O'Brien RT, Biller DS. Dental imaging. In: Gaughan EM, DeBowes RM, eds. The Veterinary Clinics of North America, Equine Practice: Dentistry. Philadelphia: WB Saunders 1998;14(2):259–271.
5. Pascoe JR. Dental radiography/radiology. Proceedings of the American Association of Equine Practitioners: 1991:99–111.
6. Park RD. Radiographic examination of the equine head. In: Honnas CM, Bertone AL, eds. The Veterinary Clinics of North America, Equine Practice: The Equine Head. Philadelphia: WB Saunders, 1993.
7. Dik KJ, Gunsser I. Atlas of diagnostic radiology of the horse: part 3: diseases of the head, neck and thorax. Philadelphia: WB Saunders, 1990.
8. O'Brien RT. Intraoral dental radiography: experimental study and clinical use in two horses and a llama. Vet Radiol Ultrasound 1996;37:412–416.
9. Baker GJ. Some aspects of equine dental radiology. Equine Vet J 1971;3:46–51.
10. Gibbs C. The equine skull: its radiological interpretation. J Am Radiol Soc 1974;15:70–78.
11. Barbee DD, Allen JR, Gavin PG. Computed tomography in horses. Vet Radiol Ultrasound 1987;28:144–1151.
12. Tietje S, Becker M, Bockenhoff G. Computed tomographic evaluation of head diseases in the horse: fifteen cases. Equine Vet J 1996;28:98–105.
13. Biller D, Myer W. Ultrasound scanning of superficial structures using an ultrasound standoff pad. Vet Radiol Ultrasound 1988;29:138–142.
14. Metcalfe MR, Tate LP, Sellett LC. Clinical use of [99m]TC-MDP scintigraphy in the equine maxilla. Veterinary Radiology 1989;30:80–87.

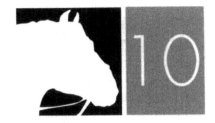

DENTAL INFECTIONS

PATRICIA PENCE AND TONY BASILE

Infections of dental tissues are relatively common in horses of all ages. Many equine primary caregivers lack the training, the equipment, or both to perform a proper dental examination. Horses may not show signs of discomfort due to dental disease, so it frequently goes unnoticed until it is advanced.

Dental sepsis is infection involving the living structures supporting the tooth: the gingiva, the alveolus, the periodontal ligament, and the tooth pulp. Dental caries pertain to a degenerative process involving demineralization of the tooth that can lead to continuous destruction of cementum, enamel, and dentin. Dental disease in the horse can originate at the gingival margin as periodontal disease, in infundibuli with abnormal cementum formation, or in the apical region of the tooth as pulpitis. Both periodontal disease and pulpitis are usually secondary to inflammatory or infectious conditions created by malocclusions, maleruption or impaction of teeth; fractures of the tooth, mandible, or maxilla; or the presence of caries. By the time dental sepsis is recognized, infection has usually invaded the pulp cavity, the periodontium, or both, necessitating salvage procedures or extraction.

This chapter will introduce the practitioner to the pathophysiology, clinical signs, and treatment options of dental infections seen in the horse.

■ ■ PATHOPHYSIOLOGY OF DENTAL INFECTIONS IN THE HORSE

The tooth is supported and nourished by the tissues surrounding the tooth—the gingiva, cementum, periodontal ligament, and alveolar bone—and by the tissue within the tooth—the pulp. The health and integrity of the tooth is at risk whenever the vitality of any of these tissues is compromised.

The gingival mucosa is tightly attached to the subcutaneous connective tissue that covers the bones of the mandible and maxilla. In the regions surrounding the teeth, the marginal gingiva depresses into the gingival sulcus and terminates as junctional epithelium. The junctional epithelium attaches to the subgingival cementum of the tooth. The periodontal ligament begins where the junctional epithelium ends. This area is constantly remodeling and forming new attachments as the tooth erupts.[1]

KEY POINT:
▶ The periodontal tissues (gingiva, cementum, periodontal ligament, and alveolar bone) undergo continuous remodeling and formation of new attachments to allow prolonged eruption of hypsodont teeth.[1]

Cementum is a calcified tissue that is similar to bone in mechanical characteristics and histological appearance. Subgingival cementum is a living tissue that receives nourishment from the periodontal vasculature.[1] The organic component of cementum is comprised primarily of collagen fibers produced by cementoblasts. Some of these collagen fibers, combined with collagen fibers produced by fibroblasts in the periodontal membrane, bridge the periodontal space to anchor the tooth to the alveolar bone.[1] These bridging bundles of collagen fibers are called Sharpey's fibers. The periodontal ligament is composed of nerves, blood vessels, and the dense bundles of connective tissue fibers that attach the tooth to the alveolar bone. These fibers suspend the tooth in the periodontal space to cushion it against the pressures of mastication by allowing a small amount of movement within the periodontal space. Pulp is composed of blood vessels, lymphatics, nerves, and connective tissue, which supply nutrition to the odontoblasts lining the pulp cavity. Odontoblasts produce dentin, a substance made up of approximately 70% hydroxyapatite crystals and 30% organic components including collagen fibers, mucopolysaccharides, and water.[1] Dentin production continues throughout the life of the tooth and leads to a gradual reduction in the size and volume of the pulp chamber.[1]

KEY POINT:
▶ The production of dentin continues throughout the life of the tooth.[1,2]

Odontoblasts produce dentin when the tooth is injured in an effort to prevent exposure of the pulp cavity. The nerves in the pulp innervate the odontoblasts and dentinal tubules. Signals transmitted when the tooth is injured cause increased production of reparative dentin in the injured area.[1,2] Dentin production decreases if the pulp is infected and ceases when the pulp dies.[3]

Reparative dentin is also produced in response to the chronic, low-grade irritation to the odontoblasts caused by the abrasion forces and repetitive pressures of mastication. This seals the pulp so that normal attrition of the occlusal surface does not open the pulp to the environment.[1-3]

Inflammation of the pulp causes edema of pulpal tissues. The restrictive confines of the pulp canal in a mature tooth create a situation in which the edema of the pulp causes compression and collapse of the microcirculation to the pulp. The result is pressure necrosis and pulp death.[3-7]

In the early stages of disease, the horse may chew more slowly and in an abnormal manner. The horse may chew on just one side or hold its head in a peculiar position. Boluses of undermasticated roughage (quids) may pack the cheeks or be expelled from the mouth.[7] Sometimes the horse will stop eating and rub its head against the manger, then resume eating. A horse with dental abnormalities may have no problem eating grass or mash but is reluctant to eat grain or hay, especially alfalfa stems. Inspection of the oral cavity may reveal abrasions or lacerations of the buccal mucosa or the lateral edges of the tongue from sharp enamel points.

PRACTICE TIP:

Abrasions of the buccal mucosa opposite the upper #11 teeth may be the only soft-tissue injury, so it is important to palpate that area on both sides of the mouth.

As disease becomes advanced, the horse may avoid having its head touched, grind its teeth, or salivate profusely while eating. There may be maxillary, facial, or mandibular swelling, with or without draining sinus tracts. A foul-smelling nasal discharge suggests sinus empyema. Long dental overgrowths may mechanically impair the normally vigorous chewing motions of the mandible. An examination of the feces will show evidence of inadequate mastication in the form of long stems and whole-grain particles. Food accumulating in the oral cavity eventually leads to gingivitis and periodontal disease. Intermittent episodes of colic, possibly related to indigestion or partial impaction, may be part of the history.

KEY POINT:

▶ Clinical signs of dental infections depend on the chronicity of the infection and on the location of the tooth.[2]

Maleruptions and Impactions

Maleruption can result from any condition that inhibits normal eruption and exfoliation of deciduous teeth. Conformation defects in which the rostral premolar teeth (the 06s) of opposing arcades do not exactly match up, i.e., one tooth projects out over the other, are common in horses.[8] The unopposed portion of tooth overgrows into a hook, which prevents rostral movement of the opposing arcade. This caudal pressure can impinge on the normal eruption of the deciduous teeth and cause them to be retained after they should have exfoliated. This can lead to two types of sequelae: maleruption or impaction of permanent teeth or a localized bacteremia of hematogenous origin in the inflamed pulp (anachoretic pulpitis).

The developing roots of the permanent teeth beneath the caps are growing and expanding against the bone of the mandible or maxilla. The expansive pressures within the growing root of the impacted tooth increase, creating inflammation and swelling of the supporting tissues. In this hyperemic state, the tooth is susceptible both to hematogenous colonization by bacteria and to trauma. The result is periapical abscess formation.

Impacted permanent teeth sometimes find a path outside the normal one to erupt. The most common maleruptions are lingual displacement of cheek teeth and caudal displacement of incisors.

■■   TREATMENT OPTIONS

Frequent dental examinations (every 2 to 3 months) of horses between the ages of $2\frac{1}{2}$ and $4\frac{1}{2}$ years will allow timely removal of deciduous teeth (caps) and identification of impacted teeth. A permanent tooth that erupts several weeks before the opposing tooth will be too long and need reduction to allow unimpeded eruption of the "late" tooth *(Fig. 10.1)*. The "late" deciduous tooth cap should be removed.

Deciduous incisors may not shed because the permanent incisor is not erupting directly beneath its deciduous counterpart. If the deciduous incisor is overdue to be

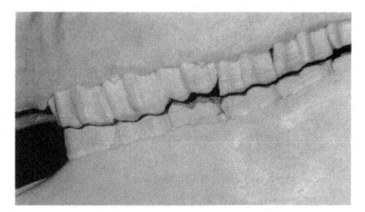

Figure 10.1 Eruption of permanent tooth #308 is impaired by the overlying deciduous tooth. The opposing permanent tooth #208 has already shed its cap and will be in wear soon. Delayed shedding of deciduous #308 puts abnormal pressure on the entire tooth, especially the expanding periapical region. If the retained deciduous tooth is not removed soon, the pressure on the apex of #308 will result in pulpitis. Another problem associated with asynchronous shedding of opposing teeth is the creation of a situation in which the early erupting tooth is always longer than its late-erupting counterpart.

shed and the presence of a permanent incisor has been established by palpation or radiography, then the deciduous incisor should be extracted. If the permanent incisor is already in the process of malerupting and is crowding or being crowded by another incisor, deciduous or permanent, trim the portions of both teeth that are contacting each other all the way to the gingival margin. Caudally displaced permanent incisors will usually realign in the incisor arcade, once the offending deciduous incisors are removed.[8]

Periapical Disease

Periapical disease is inflammation or infection of the tissues associated with the tooth apex. It can occur as an extension of pulpal inflammation, hematogenous delivery of bacteria, periodontal disease, or trauma.[3,7,9] Apical infections of the upper cheek teeth appear to arise at the clinical crown, and infections of the lower cheek teeth most commonly begin in the periapical region.[6] Abscess formation occurs when bacteria invade and colonize the unhealthy tissues. As the infection progresses, the inflammation and suppuration follow the path of least resistance along the periapical structures, causing destruction of the periodontal ligament and alveolar bone lysis.[10]

The permanent #07s or #08s are the most common teeth to succumb to periapical infections.[2,11] Periapical abscesses of mandibular teeth are most commonly seen in horses aged 3 to 6 years.[11] Maxillary periapical abscesses are more common in horses older than 6 years.[2,11,12]

Clinical signs depend on chronicity of infection and the location of the tooth involved.[2] Mandibular tooth root abscesses are usually accompanied by swelling along the ventral jaw and fistula formation. Sometimes the infection travels dorsally and breaks out into the mouth, which causes a foul odor on the breath. The signs of maxillary tooth root abscesses depend on whether the roots and reserve crown of the affected teeth erupt into the paranasal sinuses. With upper teeth #06, 07, and 08, apical osteitis, maxillary facial swelling, and fistula formation are the most common signs. The roots and reserve crowns of teeth #09 and 10 lie within the rostral maxillary sinus, and those of the #11s lie in the caudal maxillary sinus in horses until their late teens to early twenties. Clinical signs of apical infection of the last three upper cheek teeth include foul-smelling discharge from the ipsilateral nostril, halitosis, and periodontal disease of tissue adjacent to the affected tooth. Epiphora may be present if the inflammatory response involves the nasolacrimal duct.[10]

Radiographic signs are those associated with chronic alveolar periostitis, i.e., periapical bone lysis, loss of the periodontal ligament, lysis of the root, and sometimes sclerosis of adjacent bone *(Fig. 10.2)*. Long-standing cases of maxillary tooth disease can present with fluid in the paranasal sinuses and calcification of soft tissues in the sinus.[13]

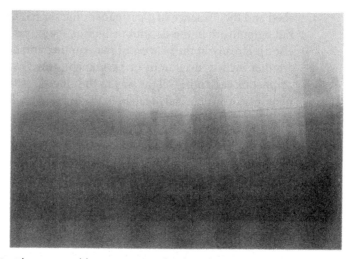

Figure 10.2   This 4-year-old mare presented with unilateral submandibular swelling. The radiograph shows extensive tooth root lipis, periapical bone lipis, and fistulous tracts leading from 307 and 308.

KEY POINT:

▶ Abscessed maxillary tooth roots are seen most often in horses over 5 years old. The teeth usually affected are maxillary #7 and 9, and occasionally #8. Mandibular root abscesses usually involve teeth #7 and 8 and are most common in horses between the ages of 3 to 6 years.[7,2,10]

■ ■   TREATMENT OPTIONS

Antibiotic therapy has been reported to be successful in treating the early stage of periapical infections in teeth with immature roots and large, open pulp canals. The pulp in these teeth is not as subject to pressure necrosis as the more-confined pulp in teeth with mature roots.[6,7,10] Conservative therapy has been more successful with mandibular than maxillary cheek teeth.[6] Curettage of affected mandibular apices has been tried with variable success.[10]

Antibiotics should be broad spectrum (procaine penicillin G 22,000–44,000 IU/kg IM every 12 hours), in combination with trimethoprim-sulfa (30–50 mg/kg orally every 12 hours) and given for 2 to 4 weeks. If *B. fragilis* is suspected, metronidazole (15–20 mg/kg orally every 12 hours) should be added.

If antibiotic therapy is unsuccessful, then the maturity of the tooth root and integrity of the supporting structures should be evaluated radiographically. If there are no other complicating factors, the root of the tooth is sufficiently mature, and the periodontal structures are still intact, then an apicoectomy can be considered. Apicoectomy procedures require appropriate equipment and operator training. At this time, this procedure has had some success in saving mandibular teeth. The success rate in maxillary teeth is much lower due to complicating anatomical issues. Maxillary teeth are intimately associated with the sinuses and other vital structures. In addition, maxillary teeth have 3 to 4 roots, whereas mandibular teeth have only 2 roots. Equine apicoectomy procedures are beyond the scope of this book and have been well described elsewhere.[14–19]

In cases in which the teeth in question have immature roots that have not responded to antibiotics, that have complicating factors that make the success of endodontic therapy unlikely, or in which endodontic therapy is not feasible, extraction is the treatment of choice. Extractions will be described in Chapter 11.

Treatment of dental-associated sinusitis requires removal of the affected tooth, debridement of the pyogenic mucosal membrane, and twice-daily lavage of the sinuses through a trephine opening.[20]

Periodontal Disease

Periodontal disease, also called alveolar periostitis, is the presence of disease in the periodontal tissues: the alveolus, cementum, periodontal ligament, and gingiva. Periodontal disease in horses has been documented in veterinary literature as early as 1905. Colyer noted in the Veterinary Record the presence of periodontal disease in 166 out of 500 skulls of horses that died in London that year.[21] Little also described periodontal disease in the horse in 1913.[22]

Periodontal disease is a chronic, progressive, septic inflammation of the periodontal structures that, if left untreated, can result in loss of alveolar bone, invasion of periapical tissues, septic pulpitis, and finally, the loss of the tooth. Periodontal disease begins as mild inflammation at the surface of the gingival margin. A transient periodontitis has been reported to be associated with the eruption of permanent teeth in young horses.[2,6] Studies of the teeth and gingiva of hundreds of skulls have shown that up to 60% of horses over the age of 15 have periodontal disease.[2,12]

Dental abnormalities that inhibit normal mastication are the most common cause of periodontal disease in the horse.[2,6] Normally, the tight arrangement of teeth in an arcade prevents food from becoming trapped between them. Very little plaque and tartar accumulate on cheek teeth that have good occlusion and normal occlusal forces.[2,6] The frictional forces of normal mastication and normal movement of food through the oral cavity contribute to oral hygiene and gingival health. Anatomical abnormalities of the teeth affect mastication by causing uneven distribution of occlusal pressure and short, choppy, mandibular motions. Uneven tooth eruption, hooks, waves, overgrown incisors, and pain from sharp dental points prevent adequate lateral excursion. In addition, hooks and ramps on corner

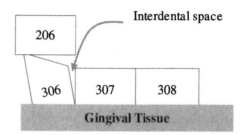

Figure 10.3 Diagram of abnormal rostral forces tilting lower second premolar rostrally. This creates a gap for food to pack in. (Illustration courtesy of Tony Basile from Proper Equine Dentistry, 2000, CD-ROM.)

cheek teeth (#06s, #11s) place abnormal rostral pressure on these teeth. This pressure eventually tips them rostrally, allowing a small interocclusal space to form (author's observation and anecdotal observations by other dental practitioners) *(Fig. 10.3)*.

The most severe periodontal disease is usually secondary to severe overgrowth of cheek teeth. Shear mouth (chronic enamel overgrowth), supernumerary caudal cheek teeth, displaced and rotated teeth (maleruptions), sagittally fractured teeth, and overgrowth of teeth into spaces left by missing teeth are conditions that impair normal mastication.[2,5] Missing teeth allow mesial and distal movement of adjacent teeth, which widens the interproximal spaces, enabling food particles to accumulate in them. Malaligned (twisted or tilted) or malformed teeth can also be associated with abnormal spaces between teeth.

Another factor contributing to periodontal disease in the horse is the shape of the reserve crown. The tooth tapers in diameter from the occlusal surface to the roots. As the reserve crown is lost to attrition, the tooth gradually narrows in width. Eventually, small gaps (diastemata) appear between the oldest teeth.[23,24] Food particles collect in these gaps, ferment, and create an inflammatory condition that eventually progresses to periodontal disease.

Diet also plays an important role in equine oral health. A diet with adequate quantities of high-quality, long-stem roughage helps prevent some abnormalities of dental wear. It has been reported that the length of the stems of the roughage dictates the extent of lateral excursion of the mandible during mastication and that horses on diets that are high in concentrates or pellets exhibit much shorter lateral strokes.[11] Reduced lateral excursion is thought to be a contributing factor to enamel overgrowth.

Other factors that can contribute to the development and progression of periodontal disease are age, general health, breed, immune status, oral trauma, and local irritants (grass awns).[23]

The inhibition of the normal movement of food through the oral cavity causes food to build up in the buccal spaces of the upper cheek teeth and lingual spaces of the lower cheek teeth.[24] These neglected boluses of food ferment, causing irritation and bacterial colonization of the gingival margins, leading to erosion of the lateral gingival margin. Without normal frictional forces to cleanse the oral cavity, plaque accumulates on the surface of the teeth. Plaque is an organic matrix composed of salivary glycoproteins, oral bacteria, and inorganic material derived from food particles. Bacterial fermentation releases compounds that cause inflammation, hyperemia, and edema of the gingiva and invasion of the gingival sulcus.[23]

The inflamed gingiva separate from the tooth, creating periodontal pockets that allow accumulation of more food and bacteria. The inflammation and infection can lead to breakdown of the periodontal attachments and loss of alveolar bone and can eventually spread distally to the tooth apex and pulp tissue *(Fig. 10.4)*.

Signs of periodontal disease vary and may depend on the severity of the disease and the pain tolerance of the individual horse. Horses with clinical disease may eat slowly and eat reduced quantities. Horses may have quids of partially chewed roughage packed in their cheeks. Quids may also be found near the area where the horse is fed. Halitosis, salivation, sensitivity to cold water, and loss of condition may be seen.

Periodontal disease in the horse has been divided into four categories based on the severity of the lesions *(Box 10.1)*.

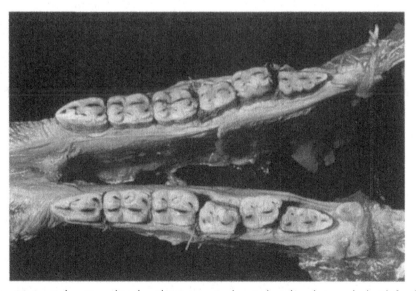

Figure 10.4 Malpositioned teeth with interproximal periodontal pockets packed with food. (Reprinted with permission from Baker GJ, Easley J, eds. Equine dentistry. Philadelphia: WB Saunders, 1998.)

BOX 10.1   CATEGORIES OF PERIODONTAL DISEASE[23]

1. Local gingivitis with hyperemia and edema.
2. Recession of gingival margin to 5 mm and periodontal pocket formation.
3. Periodontitis with loss of gum.
4. Gross periodontal pocketing, lysis of alveolar bone, loosening of bone support.

■ ■ TREATMENT OPTIONS

Periodontal disease in the horse appears to be reversible to some extent due to the continuous remodeling of the periodontium to accommodate prolonged eruption. The equine periodontium accommodates the prolonged eruption of reserve crown by the continuous development of new periodontal fibers.[6] Currently, treatment involves correcting the occlusal abnormalities, extracting very loose or diseased teeth, removing tartar, cleaning out periodontal pockets, and packing pockets with an antibiotic gel. Instruments needed to clean periodontal pockets include a variety of dental picks, scalers, and rinsing equipment.

Start by removing the food packed in the pocket with a dental pick. Gently pick out the pocket, trying not to cause further soft-tissue damage and excess bleeding. Tartar can be removed manually using human dental instruments or an ultrasonic scaler. As with other species, horses can have tartar accumulate below the gumline as well as above it. This subgingival tartar is more likely to contribute to periodontal disease and should be removed if possible. The vibrating tip of the ultrasonic scaler can scale off tartar in deep periodontal pockets that would be difficult to reach with hand instruments. Follow the scaling procedures by rinsing out the pocket thoroughly. The pulsating stream created by an oral cleansing unit designed for home use is an efficient way to thoroughly clean the pocket. It is not known whether polishing teeth after scaling will reduce tartar buildup in horses.

After thoroughly cleaning the pocket, rinse it with a diluted antiseptic, such as chlorhexidine. Dry the pocket with sterile gauze or compressed air. Finally, infuse the pocket and gingival margins with Pharmacia Doxyrobe gel. Doxyrobe gel is a product that is specifically designed for the treatment of periodontal disease. It is a gel-like substance that contains an antibiotic. The gel hardens to a rubbery consistency, and antibiotic is released over a period of weeks.

Recheck and retreat the pocket at intervals of 14 days until the pocket has healed. In cases in which there is extensive alveolar bone loss, there may be significant gingival recession that is most likely irreversible. However, gingival recession is preferable to a bacteria-collecting periodontal pocket.

PRACTICE TIP:

A portable oral irrigation unit can be used to thoroughly clean perio-pockets. A can of compressed air with an extension tip can be used to dry perio-pockets before application of antibiotic gel.

Deep periodontal pockets may result in infection of the periapical tissues, including the pulp. Inflammation and edema of tissue at the root apex extends into the pulp canal and causes hypoxia and pressure necrosis of the pulp. The end result is a dead tooth. Without the support of the alveolar attachments, the tooth becomes loose and functionless in its socket. If the tooth is excessively loose, it should be extracted.

Dental Caries

Caries is the disease of the calcified tissues of the teeth characterized by demineralization of the inorganic components and decay of the organic components.

There has been much discussion regarding the etiology of dental caries in humans, and numerous theories have been proposed to explain this pathological condition of the teeth. Scientific evidence suggests a relationship between carbohydrates, oral microorganism, and acids in the formation of dental caries.[25,26] Some equine diets are made more palatable by incorporating cariogenic foods (sweet feeds), such as molasses and sweet potato by-products. Oral bacteria and the sugars in these feeds become incorporated in the plaque covering the exposed crowns. Bacterial fermentation can occur and produce acids that dissolve the surface cementum. These lesions are most obvious on the labial surface of incisor teeth *(Fig. 10.5)*.

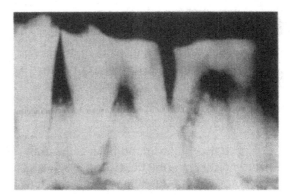

Figure 10.5 Radiologic appearance of grade IV periodontitis with loss of alveolar bone. (Reprinted with permission from Baker GJ, Easley J, eds. Equine dentistry. Philadelphia: WB Saunders, 1998.)

BOX 10.2
Categories of Dental Caries in the Horse[28]

1. Caries of cement from the occlusal surface.
2. Caries of peripheral cement *(Fig. 10.6)*.
3. Caries of root cement originating from purulent periodontitis *(Fig. 10.7)*.
4. Caries from an open pulp cavity.

PRACTICE TIP:

Although no studies have shown a reduction in caries in horses that are not fed sweet feeds, it may be wise to discourage feeding diets high in molasses until there is evidence that these diets do not significantly contribute to caries formation.

Dental caries of the occlusal surface are often associated with hypoplastic infundibula (infundibula that are not adequately filled with cementum). The infundibula are enamel invaginations found in the incisors and maxillary cheek teeth. Cementum is deposited with the infundibulum during the development of the tooth by cementoblasts nourished by the blood supply associated with the dental sac. After the tooth erupts, the cementum loses its blood supply and becomes inert mineralized tissue.[1] Infundibular necrosis, a term previously used to describe carious lesions of the infundibulum, is not appropriate because it implies the death of living tissue. Infundibula that are not adequately filled with cementum become packed with food and bacteria. Fermentation and acid production within the infundibulum lead to decalcification of the cementum, enamel, and dentin. Infundibular decay or caries is a more accurate description of these lesions. Localized caries are common in the infundibula of the horse and are usually benign.[24] One study reported caries of the infundibular cement in 43% of otherwise normal maxillary cheek teeth.[27] Although this is a relatively important source of caries in the horse, hypoplastic infundibula do not always develop caries. Future research may identify other factors that are involved.

Baker describes four types of dental caries in the horse *(Box 10.2)* and offers a system for grading caries by severity *(Box 10.3)*.

BOX 10.3
Grades of Severity[28]

1. Caries of the infundibular cementum *(Fig 10.7)*.
2. Caries of infundibular cementum and surrounding enamel *(Fig 10.8)*.
3. Caries of infundibular cementum, enamel, and dentin.
4. Splitting of the tooth as a result of caries *(Fig 10.9)*.
5. Loss of the tooth due to caries.

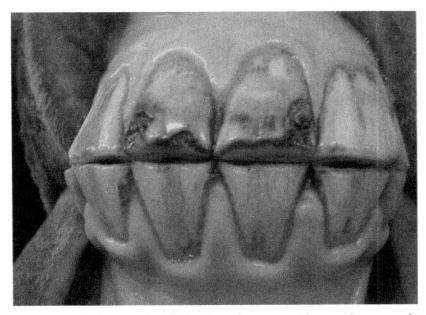

Figure 10.6   Carious lesion on the labial surface of an incisor. (Photograph courtesy of Tony Basile from the Future of Equine Dentistry, 2000, CD-ROM.)

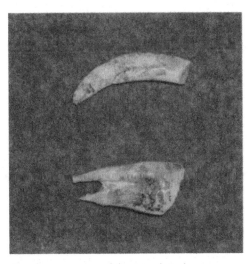

Figure 10.7   The discolored appearance of these teeth is due to exposure to acids in the purulent exudate associated with severe periodontitis. The pits in the surface are superficial caries in the cementum. These teeth were very loose and easily extracted.

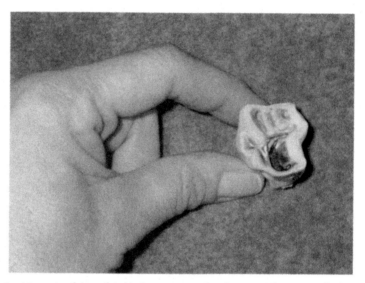

Figure 10.8   Necrosis of the infundibular cementum and surrounding enamel. The enamel is darkened, and there is 3 mm pitting in the infundibulum. Food was packed in the infundibulum.

■ ■   TREATMENT OF DENTAL CARIES

Treating caries is not currently a routine component of equine dentistry. Although there is not sufficient scientific data to prove the significance of all carious conditions in the horse, it is apparent that caries of the infundibulum can progress until the pulp is penetrated. Clinical experience has shown that cleaning

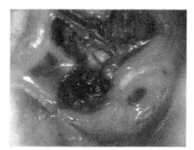

Figure 10.9   Necrosis of the infundibular cementum, surrounding enamel, and dentine. Pitting was in excess of 6 mm, the infundibulum was packed with food, and a foul odor was present. (Photo taken with intra-oral camera by Tony Basile.)

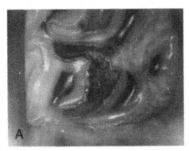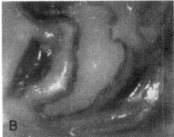

Figure 10.10 Before and after appearance of maxillary cheek tooth after the necrotic infundibulum was debrided, sterilized, and filled. (Photo taken with intra-oral camera by Tony Basile.)

and filling these areas with a composite may arrest the decomposition of the tooth *(Fig. 10.10)*.[15,29] Each carious lesion must be approached as a unique situation and evaluated for severity of decomposition of the infundibular enamel. Not every cavity needs to be filled. However, for a filling to save the tooth, the degenerated tooth material must be debrided and the tooth sterilized and filled before the lesion has advanced to the point that bacteria can traverse the dentinal tubules to the pulp. An excellent light source with magnification is needed to evaluate caries. This can be accomplished with a flexible or rigid endoscope, or an intra-oral camera.

Equi-Dent Technologies offers an Equine Composite Restoration Kit, which includes video instructions, and the equipment and supplies needed to debride and fill equine caries *(Box 10.4)*.

BOX 10.4 EQUINE COMPOSITE RESTORATION KIT
Equi-Dent Technologies, P.O. Box 5877, Sparks, NV 89432
775-358-6695

1. Equine composite restoration instructional video.
2. Medidenta Air-Abrasion Unit. Used by human dentists for "drill-less" removal of decayed dental tissue.
3. Demitron 300 Curing Light. Used to cure adhesive and to harden the composite.
4. Composite System. Contains light-activated composite, acid etchant, Optibond adhesive, and applicators.
5. Hand instruments. Condensor/spreader, spatula, explorer, burnisher, dental mirror, and irrigation syringe.

KEY POINT:

▶ As more practitioners evaluate, treat, and share results of treatment of carious lesions in equine teeth, we will have more information on the success rate and practicality of the techniques described.

Iatrogenic Cellulitis and Osteomyelitis

Trauma to the oral mucosa or bone, either intentionally (as in extractions) or unintentionally, can result in infections of the soft tissue or bone. Common places for trauma to occur are the tissue associated with the caudal cheek teeth (#11s), the gingiva and palate associated with the rostral cheek teeth (#06s), the tongue, and the buccal mucosa.

The oral cavity behind the #11s can be difficult to visualize when dental instruments are in place. When using carbide burrs, it is important to have the back of the mouth well lit and to stop burring immediately if the burr slips off the tooth or if copious bleeding occurs. An assistant should hold the tongue to the side when using molar cutters and help the dentist make sure that the handles of the cutters are parallel with the arcade before cutting is attempted. Holding the handles too high can result in cutting off an excessive amount of tooth or even cutting into the curvature of the mandible.

Trauma to the gingiva on either side of the tooth can occur when putting in bit seats. The tongue and buccal mucosa must be retracted or protected with a burr guard. When working on the medial side of the bit seat, push the palate tissue away with a finger.

A horse that is not adequately sedated can sustain severe injury to the tongue when it tries to push the burring instrument out of its mouth with its tongue.

Do not hesitate to administer broad-spectrum antibiotics and anti-inflammatory medication if the soft tissue is severely abraded. If a deep wound is created in the tongue, curvature of the mandible, or the back of the mouth, antibiotics should be continued for 3 to 5 days. Tetanus prophylaxis should be administered if the horse is not current or if the vaccination status is unknown.

Fractures of the Mandible, Maxilla, or Teeth

Fractures of the mandible, maxilla, or teeth may be the source of acute dental sepsis if the pulp or periapical tissues are exposed to bacterial contamination. Kicks, collisions, and falls may result in these types of injuries. Dental and facial fractures are seen in polo ponies struck by a polo mallet or ball. Trapping the mandible in the bars of a stall gate, panel, or fence is a fairly common accident in horses that results in the fracture of one or both sides of the mandible. Presumably, long canine teeth can also contribute to mandibular entrapment.

Clinical signs of fractures vary with the fracture site. Fractures of the mandibular or maxillary incisive bone or avulsion of incisors may not be visible without parting the lips unless the teeth are dramatically displaced. These wounds are usually filled with decomposing feed, blood clots, and devitalized tissue. The horse may salivate excessively and have a foul odor to the mouth. Fractures at the level of the interdental space of the mandible are usually bilateral and may result in instability of the rostral mandible. Fractures involving the interdental space of the maxilla are not as common as those of the mandible. Soft-tissue swelling, hemorrhage from the oral cavity, malalignment of teeth, and difficulty eating may be seen. Oral examination may show mucosal laceration and crepitation. Horses with caudal mandibular fractures may show signs of soft-tissue swelling, malalignment of cheek teeth, and dysphagia.

Fractures of the temporomandibular joint are rare. Horses with fractures in this area show signs of soft-tissue swelling, painful response to palpation, unwillingness to open the mouth, rostral or caudal displacement of the mandible, and malalignment of the cheek teeth.

Fractures of the mandible or maxilla that involve cheek teeth are the most serious in terms of malocclusion and tooth loss due to loss of alveolar support or infection. Inadequate fracture stabilization or alignment may lead to severe malocclusion and temporomandibular joint problems. Even seemingly minor fractures involving the alveolar socket can become contaminated with oral bacteria and lead to septic periodontitis and pulpitis.

Radiography should be used when fractures of the interdental space, caudal mandible, or temporomandibular joint are suspected. Lateral, oblique, and dorsoventral views should be taken to highlight the fracture and identify whether the fracture is comminuted and if teeth are involved. Radiography is not usually needed for fractures involving the incisors and the incisive bones.

Fractures of individual teeth can be the result of degenerative pathology or trauma. Teeth weakened by caries can eventually crack, exposing the pulp to oral bacteria. This most commonly occurs in maxillary cheek teeth, partially due to their susceptibility to caries of the infundibula. The affected tooth usually fractures sagittally along the decayed infundibulum. Food tends to pack in between the fracture pieces, displacing them buccally and/or lingually into the soft tissues. Trauma to the buccal mucosa or tongue may be present if this occurs. In long-standing cases, focal overgrowth of the opposing tooth may be present.[30]

Idiopathic, i.e., not associated with trauma or decay, slab fractures of cheek teeth have also been reported.[30] Slab fractures of cheek teeth seldom involve the pulp cavity. Treatment is usually limited to removal of the fractured pieces of tooth, which may still have gingival attachments.

Iatrogenic pulp exposure can occur if teeth are fractured when they are being reduced with percussion cutters or molar cutters. The percussion cutter can slip as the cutting blow is delivered, causing the tooth to shear into the pulp or to shatter. Using molar cutters that are too small for the tooth applies an uneven scissors pressure on the tooth, which can cause it to shatter instead of shear off. Even if the tooth is not fractured, overgrown teeth may have pulp extending into the part of the crown that is being reduced. If the pulp or periapical tissues are exposed, an acute septic pulpitis can be the result.

■ ■ TREATMENT OPTIONS

The treatment described here will be limited to first aid, stabilization of partially avulsed incisors, and tooth capping. Fracture fixation is beyond the scope of this book and has been well described by other authors.[31–34]

The initial treatment of fractures of the mandible or maxilla involves cleaning and debriding fractures that open into the oral cavity. Sedate the horse and support the head with a headstand or suspend the head from a dental halter if the fracture is limited to the incisors or premaxilla. Use of a full-mouth speculum may be contraindicated, but a wedge speculum may be used to improve access if the fracture is limited to the incisive bones. Flush out food and blood clots with a dose syringe, and inspect the wound. Debride devitalized tissue, and remove small bone fragments. Rinse frequently with dilute povidone iodine or chlorhexidine. Many times, fractures of the mandible are nondisplaced, and surgical fixation may not be necessary.[5,30]

Partially avulsed incisors can frequently be tapped back into the alveolus and stabilized with cerclage wire if necessary. The exact configuration of the wire is dependent on the fracture. Holes are drilled between the incisors using a Steinman pin or a 3.2 mm drill bit. A 14-gage or 16-gage needle can sometimes be used successfully to drill the holes if no other equipment is available and will facilitate guiding the wire through the holes regardless of the type of drill used *(Fig. 10.11)*. Stainless steel cerclage wire, 1.2 mm or larger, is fed through the holes. Align the incisive surfaces of the teeth and recheck them as you tighten the wire. Do not begin to tighten the wire until you have taken all of the slack out of it. Any kinks or bends put into the wire may make tightening more difficult. Pull the wire ends straight out away from the teeth toward the lips, and make the first twist as close to the gingiva as possible. Make the wire twists as even as possible, and tighten with needle holders or pliers. Cut the wire and bend it down onto the gingiva.[30–32]

Completely avulsed incisors are not usually salvageable; however, they can always be removed later if the tooth becomes infected. If the injury is fresh and the tooth is not dried out, try to save it. Remove blood clots and debris from the alveolus, and thoroughly rinse the alveolus and the tooth with dilute antiseptic. Fill the alveolus with penicillin and gentamicin. Carefully tap the tooth into place and stabilize with cerclage wire. Suture the lacerated gingiva associated with the tooth using an absorbable monofilament suture. Prescribe broad-spectrum antibiotics for 10 days to 2 weeks and anti-inflammatory medication for 5 to 7 days. The horse

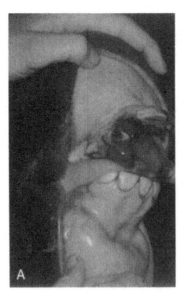

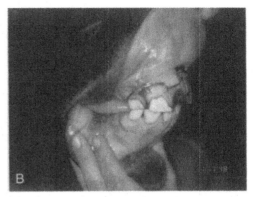

Figure 10.11 A. Partial avulsion of the incisors. B. The wound was cleared and flushed with dilute betadine. The incisors were tapped back into position and wired in place for stabilization using 16-gauge needles. (Reprinted with permission from Tony Basile, The Future of Equine Dentistry, 2000, CD-ROM.)

should be confined and fed hay (and concentrates if necessary) for 4 to 6 weeks to prevent stress on the incisors.

Teeth that are fractured into the pulp either by trauma or iatrogenically should be evaluated for the extent of pulp exposure. Remove loose pieces of crown, and rinse with dilute antiseptic. If the fracture does not extend below the gingival margin, a partial pulpotomy and pulp-capping procedure can be done.[15]

Debride devitalized pulp tissue with a spoon curette using an operative loupe for magnification. Hemorrhage must be controlled and the tooth surface dried before applying a pulp cap. Rinse the area with saline, adding epinephrine to it, and apply a pressure pack if necessary. After hemorrhage has been stopped, air-dry the tooth and etch the surface in which the cap is to be attached to. Wash and dry the tooth, then sterilize the surface with 2.5% sodium hydroxide and apply a dental adhesive made for restorative procedures. Mix calcium hydroxide (Pulpdent, Henry Schein Inc., 5 Harbor Park Dr., Port Washington, New York) or dental resin (Renamel Restorative System, Cosmedent, Inc., 5419 North Sheridan Rd., Chicago, IL 60640, 1-800-621-6729) according to the instructions and apply to the tooth as directed *(Fig. 10.12)*.

It is important that the tooth be kept out of occlusion for at least 3 months so that the fracture can be sealed with reparative dentin before the tooth is put into wear. This can be accomplished by reducing the occlusal surface of the opposing tooth.

Prescribe broad-spectrum antibiotics for a week to 10 days, anti-inflammatory medication for 5 to 7 days, and recheck the horse in 2 weeks. Look for signs of inflammation and swelling in the tooth root area of the affected tooth. If the tooth shows signs of infection, radiograph the periapical structures and evaluate the extent of infection. If there is widening of the periodontal space suggesting periapical sepsis, then the tooth will need to be extracted.

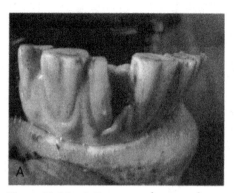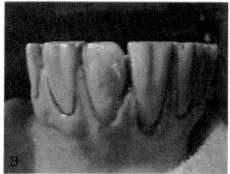

Figure 10.12   A. Transverse fracture of an incisor that entered the pulp. **B.** Appearance of the fractured incisor after restorative pulp capping with Renamel. (Photos by Tony Basile.) (Reprinted with permission from Tony Basile, The Future of Equine Dentistry, 2000, CD-ROM.)

Acknowledgments.   Special thanks to David Klugh and Randi Brannen for reviewing the earlier versions of this chapter.

■ ■   REFERENCES

1. Dixon PM. Dental anatomy. In: Baker GJ, Easley J, eds. Equine Dentistry. Philadelphia: WB Saunders, 1999.
2. Baker GJ. Dental decay and endodontic disease. In: Baker GJ, Easley JE, eds. Equine Dentistry. Philadelphia: WB Saunders, 1998:79–84.
3. Harvey CE, Emily PP. Small Animal Dentistry. St. Louis: Mosby-Year Book, 1994: 157–213.
4. Stanley HR, White CL, McCray L. The rate of tertiary (reparative dentine) formation in the human tooth. Oral Surg Oral Med Oral Pathol. 1966:180–189.
5. Lane JG. A review of dental disorders of the horse, their treatment and possible fresh approaches to management. Equine Vet Educ 1994;6:13–21.
6. Dixon PM. Dental disease. In: Robinson NE, ed. Current Therapy in Equine Medicine. 4th ed. Philadelphia: WB Saunders, 1997:149–153.
7. Uhlinger C. Survey of selected dental abnormalities in 233 horses. In: Proceedings of the 33rd Annual Convention of the American Association of Equine Practitioners. New Orleans, 1987:577–583.
8. Dixon PM, Tremaine WH, Pickles K, Kuhns L, et al. Equine dental disease part 1: a long-term study of 400 cases: disorders of the incisor, canine, and first premolar teeth. Equine Vet J 1999;31:369–377.

9. Mueller PO, Lowder MQ. Dental sepsis. Vet Clin North Am Equine Pract 1998; 14:349–363.

10. Dixon PM, Tremaine WH, Pickles K, Kuhns L, et al. Equine dental disease part 4: a long-term study of 400 cases: apical infections of cheek teeth. Equine Vet J 2000;32:182–194.

11. Easley JE, Caddel LB. Recognition and management of the diseased equine tooth. Proceedings of the 37th Annual AAEP Convention, 1991.

12. Baker GJ, Diseases of the teeth. In: Colahan PT, Mayhew IG, Merritt AM, et al., eds. Equine medicine and surgery. 4th ed. Goleta CA: American Veterinary Publishers, 1991:568.

13. Gibbs C. Dental imaging. In: Baker GJ, Easely J, eds. Equine Dentistry. Philadelphia: WB Saunders, 1998:156–162.

14. Garcia F, Sanroman, Llonens MP. Endodontics in the horse: an experimental study. J Am Vet Med Assoc 1990;37:205–214.

15. Baker GJ. Endodontic therapy. Equine Dentistry. Philadelphia: WB Saunders, 1999:250.

16. Baker GJ, Kirkland DK. Endodontic therapy in the horse. Proceedings of the 38th Annual Meeting of the American Association of Equine Practitioners, 1992:329–335.

17. Dixon PM. Dental extraction and endodontic techniques in horses. Compend Contin Educ Pract Vet 1997;19:628–638.

18. Wiggs RB, Lobprise H. Basic endodontic therapy. In: Wiggs RB, Lobprise H, eds. Veterinary Dentistry Principles and Practice. Philadelphia: Lippincott-Raven, 1997:280–328.

19. Zetner K. Equine apicoectomy. In: Proceedings of the American Dental College Meeting. New Orleans: American Veterinary Dental College, 1989.

20. Henning GE, Steckel RR. Diseases of the oral cavity and esophagus. In: Kobluk CN, Ames TR, Geor RJ, eds. The Horse: Diseases and Clinical Management. Philadelphia: WB Saunders, 1995:287–308.

21. Colyer JF. A note on dental diseases in horses. Vet Rec 1905:211–212.

22. Little WM. Periodontal disease in the horse. J Comp Pathol 1913;24:240–249.

23. Baker GJ. Abnormalities of development and eruption. In: Baker GJ, Easley J, eds. Equine Dentistry. Philadelphia: WB Saunders, 1998.

24. Dixon PM, Tremaine WH, Pickles K, Kuhns L, et al. Equine dental disease part 2: a long-term study of 400 cases: disorders of development and eruption and variations in position of the cheek teeth. Equine Vet J 1999;31:519–528.

25. Bunting RW. Studies of the relation of *Bacillus acidophilus* to dental caries. J Dent Res 1928;8:222–229.

26. Fitzgerald RJ, Jordan HV, Stanley HR. Experimental caries and gingival pathologic changes in the gnotobiotic rat. J Dent Res 1960;39:923–930.

27. Baker GJ. Some aspects of equine dental decay. Equine Vet J 1974;6:127–130.

28. Baker GJ. A study of dental disease in the horse, PhD thesis, University of Glasgow, 1979.

29. Swanstrom OG, Wallford HA. Prosthetic filling of a cement defect in premolar tooth necrosis in a horse. Vet Med Small Anim Clin 1977:1475–1477.

30. Dixon PM, Tremaine WH, Pickles K, Kuhns L, et al. Equine dental disease part 3: a long-term study of 400 cases: disorders of wear, traumatic damage and idiopathic fractures, tumours, and miscellaneous disorders of the cheek teeth. Equine Vet J 2000; 32:9–18.

31. Henning RW, Beard WL, Schneider RK, Bramlage LR, et al. Fractures of the rostral portion of the mandible and maxilla in horses: 89 cases. 1979–1997 J Am Vet Med Assoc 1999;214:1648–1652.
32. Monin T. Tension band repair of equine mandibular fractures. J Equine Med Surg 1977;1:325.
33. Stashak TS. Wound management and reconstructive surgery of the head region. In: Equine Wound Management. Philadelphia: Lea & Febiger, 1991:116–119.
34. Ragle, CA. Head trauma. In: The Equine Head. Veterinary Clinics of North America, Philadelphia: WB Saunders, 1993;9(1).

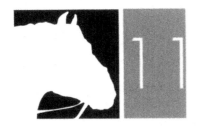

EXTRACTIONS

PATRICIA PENCE

The goal of modern equine dentistry is the preservation of teeth. In spite of advances designed to improve the dental health of the horse, extractions are still an important component of equine dentistry. Extraction is indicated for a variety of reasons, including removal of retained deciduous incisors, removal of wolf teeth, severe trauma and pulp exposure to otherwise healthy teeth, removal of diseased teeth when other efforts of management have either failed or are not feasible due to cost or lack of expertise, and removal of exceptionally loose teeth.

Client communication is critical before proceeding to remove teeth, especially in young to middle-aged horses. The client must understand that the dental needs of a horse that has had teeth extracted cannot be ignored or forgotten. Once a tooth or teeth are removed from the arcade, the dynamics of occlusion are changed forever. The adjacent teeth will drift toward the space the tooth once occupied, which will eventually result in the formation of diastema (interdental gaps) between other teeth in the arcade. Secondary periodontal disease created by food packing in the diastema and overgrowth of the now unopposed tooth in the opposite arcade will have to be managed on a regular basis. If repulsion techniques are used, the client must be informed that complications and repeat surgical procedures are not uncommon. The emphasis in this chapter will be on the intra-oral method of extraction. Repulsion techniques will be presented.

KEY POINT:
- ▶ The importance of client understanding and commitment to the long-term management of the dental needs of a horse in which teeth are extracted cannot be overemphasized.

■ ■ CONTRAINDICATIONS TO TOOTH REMOVAL

Extraction should be postponed if acute cellulitis or stomatitis is present, or if there is infection or inflammation elsewhere in the horse, until those problems are resolved. Extraction of diseased teeth will create a transient bacteriemia, which may lead to complications of other pathological conditions.[1–4] In addition, extractions, especially of diseased teeth, should not be performed at the same time as an elective surgery. The inconvenience to the client or the cost of the additional sedation, anesthesia, antibiotics, surgical suite, etc. created by performing separate procedures will seem inconsequential if severe complications arise from infection at the other surgical site.

> ### KEY POINT:
> ▶ Broad-spectrum antibiotics should be given before dental procedures, especially extractions, to horses that have infected tooth roots or periodontal disease. Geriatric horses, which may have undiagnosed Cushing's disease, should also be given antibiotics prior to these procedures. Tetanus prophylaxis should also be considered, based on the last time the horse had a booster.

Preoperative Considerations

All aspects of the procedure, including client education, postoperative care, and future therapy, should be worked out before the extraction itself is scheduled. Equipment should be assembled to ensure that nothing is missing or broken.

Other preoperative considerations include deciding on the best method to remove the tooth. The method used will depend on the location of the tooth to be removed, the age of the horse, the amount and condition of the exposed crown of the tooth to be removed, and the presence of other health issues.

Incisors are readily accessible and usually present no obstacle to removal in the standing, sedated patient. Caudal cheek teeth are a challenge regardless of technique used because space in that area of the mouth, near the *hinge*, is so limited. There is a considerable amount of unexposed crown in young horses and, unless there is extensive periodontal disease, the alveolar attachments will be quite secure. Teeth that are fractured transversely, close to the gingival margin, or longitudinally deep into the alveolus may be impossible to extract orally. Older horses, in which a standing procedure is to be performed, may not be able to lock their stay apparatus and may require torso support to prevent them from lying down.

Preoperative radiographs should be taken and carefully studied to positively identify the tooth involved prior to extraction. Even with the aid of radiographs, it is still possible to pull the wrong tooth if the position of the root relative to the crown is not mapped out. Due to the caudal curvature and the length of the reserve crown, the apex of the root is much more caudally positioned in younger mature horses.[5] As the tooth erupts, it is positioned more rostrally.

Depending on the age and physical condition of the horse, a thorough physical examination and a blood chemistry and CBC should be performed. A clotting profile should be considered also. If abnormalities are found that may complicate the procedure, such as profound anemia, hypoproteinemia, or leukocytosis, they should be addressed and corrected before subjecting the horse to the stress of an extraction. Horses with a high white cell count and a heart murmur should have a sonographic evaluation of the heart to check for bacterial endocarditis.

■ ■   **EXTRACTING INCISORS**

Permanent incisors rarely need extraction. Abnormal or supernumerary teeth that are causing pain or interfering with mastication can usually be cut or ground out of the way. Traumatic injury to incisors may necessitate removal of severely damaged or infected teeth. In cases of partial avulsion, all attempts should be made to save the teeth if the teeth themselves are intact. The injured area should be cleaned, debrided, and flushed with dilute antiseptic solution. The teeth should be tapped back into the alveolus and wired in place if necessary. Due to their inquisitive nature, these injuries are more common in young horses. The wide pulp canal of incisors in younger horses is also more forgiving of trauma than in older horses.

The presence of retained deciduous incisors is relatively common in young horses and may result in the maleruption of the permanent teeth associated with them. The short simple roots of deciduous teeth make them relatively easy to remove. Use a half-moon elevator or an orthopedic chisel to separate the root from its alveolar and mucosal attachments. It may be necessary in some cases to make a sharp incision over the root with a scalpel to obtain adequate exposure. Elevate the root, being careful to remove all of it. Rinse the surgery site with dilute antiseptic, and leave it open to heal by granulation.

Permanent incisors that require extraction are occasionally seen in horses as a sequela to trauma. An incisor with a longitudinal fracture more than a few hours old that penetrates the pulp deep into the alveolar socket will inevitably succumb to infection. If the fracture has occurred within the past 5 to 6 hours, there is a chance that the incisor can be saved by performing a partial pulpotomy and capping procedure (see Chapter 10, Dental Infections).

To remove an incisor in which the periodontal attachments are secure requires preoperative consideration of the length and curvature of the incisor, as well as its close association with the reserve crown and roots of adjacent teeth. This procedure can be done in the standing horse using a local anesthetic and sedation. Preopera-

---

BOX 11.1   EQUIPMENT NEEDED FOR ORAL EXTRACTION OF CHEEK TEETH

Rigid dental halter that can be suspended from the noseband
Full-mouth speculum
Molar spreaders
Molar forceps (extractors) appropriate for the size of tooth
Dental fulcrum and/or wooden blocks for fulcrums
Osteotome and mallet
Pointed dental pick
Root fragment forceps
Angled or curved rongeurs
Curettes
Compound-action D-head molar cutter
Portable x-ray and cassettes
Socket-packing material

---

tive antibiotics, anti-inflammatory medication, and tetanus prophylaxis are advised. The equipment required is listed in *Box 11.1*.

Incise the mucosa over the tooth longitudinally from the labial-gingival junction to the gingival margin of the tooth. Make the incision deep enough to penetrate through the mucosa and as deeply into the bone as possible. Use a ¼-inch-wide osteotome or stainless steel chisel to remove the overlying alveolar bone over the entire length of the tooth. Do not expose the reserve crown or roots of the adjacent teeth. Once the entire tooth is exposed, carefully elevate the tooth with the chisel or dental elevators by breaking down the periosteal attachments along the lateral and ventral sides of the tooth. Remove the tooth with incisor extraction forceps and flush the socket with dilute antiseptic. Excise the loose gingival flaps, and leave the wound open to drain and fill in with granulation tissue.

■ ■ EXTRACTING CANINES

Canine teeth may have to be extracted if pulp exposure from accidental trauma or overenthusiastic reduction of the crown results in pulp infection. Mandibular fractures in the interdental space can result in osteomyelitis that extends to the canine tooth *(Fig. 11.1)*. Similar to incisors and cheek teeth, there is much more tooth below the gingival margin than there is above it, so extraction is a surgical procedure. Canine teeth are more deeply embedded in the mandible than incisors and are more difficult to extract.

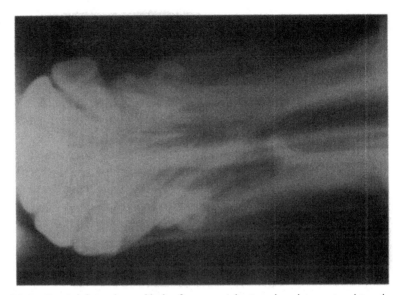

Figure 11.1 Septic bilateral mandibular fracture at the interdental space involving the canine teeth.

The practitioner should be prepared to use a general anesthetic, although canine tooth extraction can be performed in the standing horse by adequately desensitizing the mental nerve and local tissues. The overlying alveolar bone is removed and the tooth elevated and extracted in the same manner as described for incisor extraction. Wound drainage is not usually a problem in upper canines. However, lower canines should have the wound edges trimmed short and the wound rinsed with antiseptic twice daily to prevent early closure of the wound and subsequent abscess formation.

PRACTICE TIP:

Canine teeth should not be extracted to disarm a horse. It is just as effective and less invasive to grind them down.

WOLF TOOTH EXTRACTION

Wolf teeth are commonly extracted because it is well known that the presence of these vestigial teeth can cause discomfort to horses that carry bits. Extracting wolf teeth is painful to the horse, so it is more humane to the horse and safer for the dentist to administer a sedative to the horse. Infiltrating the surrounding gingiva with lidocaine is also recommended for the comfort of the horse. Using lidocaine in which epinephrine has been added will reduce bleeding.

The gingiva surrounding the wolf tooth must be elevated with a dental elevator before elevating the tooth. A round or cone-tipped Burgess elevator can be used to cut the gingiva in one quick twist; however, there is not always enough room for this elevator to fit between the wolf tooth and the first premolar. A half-moon elevator or a small canine dental elevator can be used if the teeth are close together. In cases of wolf teeth that are tight against the first premolar, the author sets a half-moon elevator or ¼-inch orthopedic chisel into the junction between the two teeth and taps the handle steadily with a small hammer until the elevator is well seated into the bone and then proceeds to elevate the root. Sometimes it is impossible to avoid breaking the root in this situation, but it does not seem to cause any problems. The owner or trainer is told that the root is still there, and the area is checked at the next dentistry to see if the root has come loose from the socket. Sometimes they can be removed easily at a later date. The broken-off root can erupt through the gingiva and present as a "new" short-rooted wolf tooth.

The entire root should be elevated on all sides prior to extraction. Once the root is elevated, the crown of the wolf tooth is grasped with dental forceps, pliers, or an old needle holder, and the tooth is removed. No postsurgical care is usually needed after removal of maxillary wolf teeth.

If no maxillary wolf teeth are visualized, the interdental space (bars) and the gingiva next to the first premolar should be palpated to make sure that there are no unerupted (blind) wolf teeth. Unerupted wolf teeth can cause the horse more discomfort than erupted wolf teeth because the gingiva over the tooth is easily irritated by the bit. Blind wolf teeth may erupt off the vertical plane, which can make removal a little more challenging. The principles are the same as for erupted wolf teeth: incise the gingiva, elevate the root, and pull out the tooth.

Occasionally, mandibular wolf teeth are seen. One author reported that they seem to be more common in some lines of standard bred horses.[6] Postsurgical drainage is more of a problem after removal of mandibular wolf teeth, so the extraction site should be lavaged and observed for signs of infection by the caretaker of the horse for several days after removal.

Instead of extracting large wolf teeth in older horses, some veterinarians prefer to reduce them to the gingival margin, because the roots of these teeth are often ankylosed to the bone.

■ ■ CHEEK TOOTH EXTRACTION

Deciding what approach to use to extract the tooth is also a preoperative consideration, if it is a cheek tooth to be extracted. Cheek teeth can be extracted by an intraoral approach or by a surgical approach.

Patient Preparation

Preoperative broad-spectrum antibiotics and anti-inflammatory medications should be given. Clean out periodontal pockets, and rinse the mouth out thoroughly with dilute antiseptic. If any other dental procedures are to be performed, such as reducing long teeth or floating, they should be done before the extraction is attempted and the mouth should be rinsed thoroughly.

The decision to use nerve blocks when extracting teeth is a personal one for the practitioner. Anecdotal reports suggest that nerve blocks vary in their ability to relieve pain—possibly due to the skill of the person performing them and possibly due to other nervous tissue supplying the anatomical structure being worked on. If a nerve block is used, a long-acting local anesthetic such as mepivacaine should be considered.

Oral Extraction of Cheek Teeth.[7,8,9] If at all possible, the intra-oral approach should be used. This technique has several advantages. It can be done in the standing horse, thereby avoiding the cost and risks associated with general anesthesia. Surgical time is usually reduced, and postoperative complications and recovery time are dramatically reduced. If more than one tooth needs to be extracted, oral extraction avoids the need for multiple surgical approaches.

Oral extractions are best performed with the horse's head suspended in a metal reinforced dental halter. Alternatively, a headstand can be used, but an assistant will have to steady it.

PRACTICE TIP:

Two assistants are needed to help the dentist perform oral extractions. Assistants can help hold the head steady; maneuver the mandible, hand instruments, sponges, etc. to the dentist; help hold molar spreaders, molar forceps, and molar cutters; and prepare the socket packing material.

After the oral cavity has been thoroughly cleansed and the tooth to be extracted has been identified, elevate the gingiva surrounding the tooth with a dental pick or ¼-inch chisel. Place the blades of the molar spreader between the affected tooth and the tooth caudal to it about ⅓ of the way down the tooth. Firmly squeeze the handles until the blades meet. Gradually work all the way down to the gingiva. Strap or tape the handles of the molar spreaders together, support the handles, and wait *(Figs. 11.2A and B)*.

KEY POINT:

▶ Oral extractions in young horses with intact periodontal ligaments can be time-consuming events. Prepare for the procedure to take a minimum of an hour, and don't try to rush; you won't be so stressed by the slow progress.

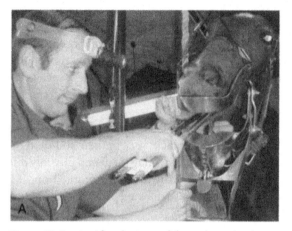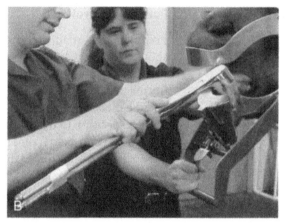

Figure 11.2 **A.** After the jaws of the molar spreaders are seated in the appropriate space, the handles are taped together, and the mandible is stabilized with the opposite hand. (Photograph courtesy of Tony Basile.) **B.** Successful oral extraction of a mandibular cheek tooth. The tip of the rostral root has been resorbed; it is not broken off.

Postoperative Care and Monitoring. Nonsteroidal anti-inflammatory medication should be administered for 3 to 5 days as deemed appropriate by the practitioner. Horses with dental infections, including periodontal disease, should be given broad-spectrum antibiotics accordingly. The horse should be monitored to make sure it is eating and drinking normally, especially the first week after the extraction.

The caretaker of the horse should be given written postoperative care instructions and should be informed to report any unusual masticatory behavior, nasal discharge, fistula formation, or foul odor coming from the mouth.

If a gauze roll or molded packing material was inserted into the alveolus, it will have to be checked to make sure it stays in place so that the alveolus does not become packed with food. Food packing in the alveolus may lead to the formation of a fistula in the ventral mandible if a mandibular tooth was removed or an oronasal fistula in the case of a maxillary tooth. If a gauze roll is used, it should be replaced every 24 to 48 hours. The shallow alveoli of geriatric horses do not need to be packed.

■ ■   **SURGICAL REMOVAL OF CHEEK TEETH**

If the affected tooth cannot be extracted orally due to advanced caries, fractures, or location, it will have to be removed surgically. Surgical extraction may be the only option to remove maxillary teeth #08 thru 11, and mandibular teeth #10 and 11 in young horses. See Table 11.1 for approaches to removal of specific cheek teeth.

Knowledge of the anatomy of cheek teeth and associated structures is vital to reduce complications. The curvature of the reserve crown and roots of cheek teeth

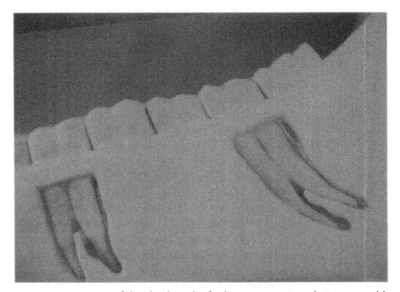

Figure 11.3 Cutaway view of the cheek teeth of a horse approximately 12 years old showing the length and curvature of the mandibular roots.

prevents easy identification of repulsion site. In addition, the location of roots is variable depending on the age of the horse *(Fig. 11.3).*[6] Roots are located more caudally in young horses and move rostrally as the horse ages and the teeth become shorter due to eruption.

In young and middle-aged horses, the roots and reserve crowns of maxillary cheek teeth #07, 08, and 09 are located in the cranial maxillary sinus. These structures are found in the caudal maxillary sinus of teeth #10 and 11. In addition to the walls of the sinuses, other vital structures that lie deep within this region are the nasolacrimal duct and the palatine artery. Maxillary teeth in geriatric horses can usually be removed orally with few complications. Surgical removal of cheek teeth has been well described by other authors.[9–11]

TABLE 11.1   Approaches for Surgical Removal of Specific Cheek Teeth[9–11]

Maxillary Teeth
#06, #07 lateral buccotomy (#08 if it does not lie within the cranial maxillary sinus)
#08 through #11 repulsion via bone flap and root resection

Mandibular teeth
#06 through #09 repulsion via trephination
#10, #11 lateral approach through masseter muscles

■ ■ REFERENCES

1. Easley J. Equine tooth removal (exodontia). In: Baker GJ, Easley J, eds. Equine dentistry. Philadelphia: WB Saunders, 1999:220–249.

2. Pascoe J. Complications of dental surgery. Proceeding of the 37th Annual Meeting of the American Association of Equine Practitioners, 1991:37, 141.

3. Conner HD, et al. Bacteremias following periodontal scaling in patients with healthy appearing gingiva. J Periodontol 1967;38:466–471.

4. Black AP, et al. Bacteremia during ultrasonic teeth cleaning and extraction in the dog. J Am Anim Hosp Assoc 1980;16:611–616.

5. Kirkland KD, Baker GJ, Maretta SM, et al. Effects of aging on the endodontic system, reserve crown and roots of equine mandibular cheek teeth. Am J Vet Res 1996;57:31–38.

6. Scrutchfield WL. Dental prophylaxis. In: Baker GJ, Easley J, eds. Equine dentistry. Philadelphia: WB Saunders, 1999:194–195.

7. Lowder MQ. Oral extraction of equine teeth. Compendium on Continuing Education for the Practicing Veterinarian 1999;21(12):1150–1157.

8. Easley J. Cheek tooth extraction: an old technique revisited. Large Animal Practice 1997:22–24.

9. Dixon PM. Dental extraction and endodontic techniques in horses. Compend Contin Educ Pract Vet 1997;19:628–637.

10. McIlwraith CW, Robertson JT. Surgery of the gastrointestinal tract. In: McIlwraith CW, Turner JT. Equine Surgery: Advanced Techniques. 2nd ed. Philadelphia: Lippincott Williams & Wilkins, 1998:289–292.

11. Lowder MQ. Tooth removal, reduction, and preservation. In: White NA, Moore JA, eds. Current Techniques in Equine Surgery and Lameness. 2nd ed. Philadelphia: WB Saunders, 1998:245–253.

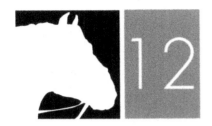

MARKETING THE EQUINE DENTAL PRACTICE

PATRICIA PENCE

The science of equine dentistry is not new to the industry of horse husbandry. As long as horses were the only means of transportation, there was a demand for men skilled in rasping sharp molar edges, cutting overlong molars or incisors, and extracting abscessed teeth. Aging horses by their teeth was a necessary art before purebred horses were registered. As the era of horse-drawn vehicles came to a close, this important aspect of equine care was left out of veterinary curriculums, resulting in several generations of veterinarians that received little to no training in equine dentistry. Now, performing more than a simple "float" is a novel idea to many horse owners. To overcome this novelty and the client reluctance that goes with trying things that are new, the equine veterinarian is faced with needing to market an aspect of horse husbandry that has existed for centuries. This chapter will present suggestions for marketing the equine dentistry service.

Marketing is a valid tool used by all professions to identify consumer wants and needs and to satisfy those wants and needs by providing the desired services and/or goods. As professionals, veterinarians are fortunate because the majority of people who own animals want to take care of them. They look to their veterinarian for guidance in selecting the best care they can afford. A veterinarian who has a good relationship with his or her clients, based on sincerity and trust, will have no problem convincing horse owners that equine dental care is not a frivolous service.

■ ■ DEVELOPING THE EQUINE DENTAL SERVICE

Developing a new service requires becoming proficient in new skills, obtaining the necessary equipment, creating records, and setting fees for the services. Just as you would not offer reproduction services if you were unfamiliar with diagnosing problems that cause reproductive failure in mares and stallions, you should first familiarize yourself with common dental problems and the use of dental equipment.

How do you go about gaining proficiency as an equine dentist? This depends on your interest level and your budget. You can participate in continuing education courses offered at veterinary colleges and at local and national veterinary meetings that include hands-on dental laboratories. You could take short courses offered by experienced equine dentists, or you could apprentice with one that lives nearby. Finally, any time you can visit and watch another equine dentist is time well spent. Because dentistry involves the use of many types of tools that can be dangerous to both the horse and the practitioner, I recommend that dental techniques either be learned in the presence of a skilled equine dentist or practiced on cadavers. Do not misrepresent your level of expertise. It is easy for the uninformed to do more harm than good with dental equipment, which opens the door for litigation opportunities.

Once you have learned to recognize common equine dental problems, understand their origin and long-term implications, and have tried enough types of equipment to know how to use them, you can begin buying your own equipment and working on client horses. I recommend you start conservatively. Buy a full-mouth speculum, a wedge speculum, a basic set of good-quality hand tools, including a couple of solid carbide float heads, a dremel motor with a flexible shaft, a diamond cut-off wheel to cut incisors, and a dremel bit to reduce protuberant upper and lower rostral cheek teeth. Any less equipment than this and you will have to spend more time in a horse's mouth than either you or the horse can stand. You can always buy more equipment if your enthusiasm for equine dentistry proves to be long term.

■ ■ EDUCATING THE HORSE-OWNING PUBLIC ABOUT EQUINE DENTAL PROBLEMS

As I said before, veterinarians are fortunate because most people who own animals want to take care of them and look to the veterinary profession for guidance about their animals' needs. Marketing the equine dental service is the process of educating the horse-owning public that regular dental care for horses is not a luxury item. It is as necessary for the good health of their horse as is food and water. The rest of this chapter will be devoted to getting the word out.

Start With Your Staff

Set aside time for your technicians, receptionists, animal assistants, and other staff members to bring their horses in to be examined *(Fig. 12.1)*. Anyone who works for you and who owns horses or has contact with other horse owners can be your best referring agent. If you've never done a full-mouth examination on your staff member's horse in their presence, do it now. Treat the staff member as though he or she is your best client by being gentle and respectful to the horse. Set aside enough time that you are not in a hurry. Sedate the horse, put in a full-mouth speculum, and perform a thorough oral examination. Explain what you are doing and why you are doing it. Have the employee horse owner visually examine his or her own horse's mouth and palpate abnormalities. Then do your best Grade A dental work, complete with bit seat, and have that person examine and palpate the mouth again. You now have a four-legged billboard and a two-legged equine dental education unit.

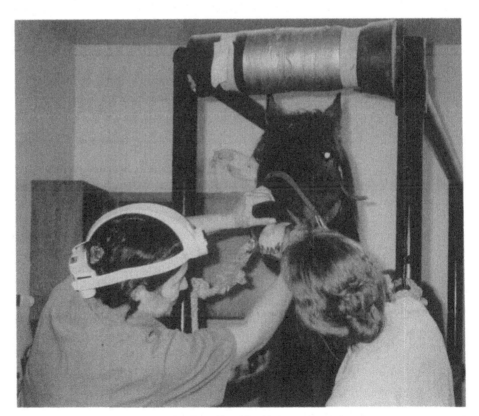

Figure 12.1 Get your staff involved by examining their horses.

Examine All Clients' Horses at Least Once a Year

Your yearly physical examination should include a full-mouth exam. Most horses need sharp enamel points floated once a year. Some horses, due to anatomical variation or performance demands, require dental work more often to stay comfortable. Include "dental examination" or "dentistry" on your vaccination reminder cards, or send separate dental examination reminder cards if you want to perform dentistry at a separate visit.

Make it a habit to check teeth no matter what the reason is for the horse's visit. It doesn't take long to do a brief examination once you become accustomed to what to look for and where to look for it (see Chapter 3 for a description of a brief examination). Check incisor alignment, molar occlusion, mouth odor, and sharpness of the points when horses come in for routine vaccinations and health certificates. If the horse is being sedated to suture a wound, you can insert a full-mouth speculum when you are finished with the wound to do a more thorough job, if it hasn't been done in the last 6 months. If you don't have time to do dental work during the appointment, you can schedule the horse for dentistry at a more convenient time.

PRACTICE TIP:

> The more often you check the mouth, the more you will reinforce in the horse owner's mind that dentistry is important.

In the Clinic

Visual reminders that emphasize the importance of equine dentistry should be displayed in areas frequented by horse clients. Commercial posters illustrating aging the horse by its teeth can be ordered from equine dental equipment catalogs. These posters can be laminated or framed and make interesting equine-oriented wall décor. You can make dentistry posters yourself, using computer-generated poster or typesetting programs, and customize them with equine clip art, photographs, or your own hand-drawn cartoons. These homemade posters, like most posters, will look more professional and be more durable if laminated or framed.

Make educational handouts available in the reception area. Both the American Association of Equine Practitioners (AAEP) and equine dental equipment dealers have pamphlets written to promote client understanding of the benefits of equine dentistry. You can also write your own handouts for a more customized version. The AAEP also has the *Official Guide to Aging the Horse* available. Pony Club and 4-H leaders as well as adults may be want to purchase this well-written booklet.

Clean, bleached horse skulls are excellent visual aids *(Fig. 12.2)*. A small collection of young, middle-aged, and old skulls illustrate how a horse's mouth and sinuses change as teeth erupt.

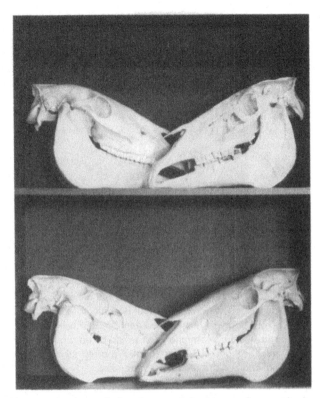

Figure 12.2 Obtain at least one skull with normal dentition and one with abnormal dentition. Skulls make it easy to explain certain abnormalities and to show how they interfere with mastication. These skulls are part of the author's collection.

KEY POINT:
▶ Skulls showing severe pathological changes such as wave mouth, uneven molar arcades, slanting incisors, long hooks, and overgrown teeth tell a story of potential pain and suffering that no oral or written reminder can equal.

In the Field

Carry a magnetic page photo album in your truck with 8 × 10 enlargements of photos you have taken of abnormal mouths you have seen and corrected. Economical 8 × 10 photocopies of color slides and 4 × 5 color prints can be made at your local full-service printing business. Photographs can be supplemented with line drawings illustrating abnormalities and their correction, as well as illustrations of aging horses by their teeth. Leave educational handouts for clients to read (*Fig. 12.3*). Most importantly, show your sincere interest in the welfare and comfort of your clients' horses. They will appreciate your concern.

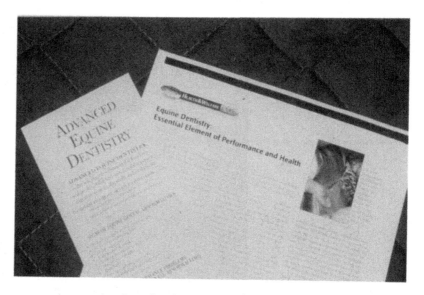

Figure 12.3 These are handouts that the author used to educate clients about modern equine dentistry. The narrow handout is printed on both sides. The text on one side has a paragraph explaining why horses need dentistry and how equine dentistry has changed. The opposite side has the information that would be on a business card and describes the author's qualifications. The other handout is a reprint of an article that the author wrote for a nationally distributed horse magazine.

Television

Television is an effective method of educating the general public about equine dentistry. Non–horse owners find the idea of doing dental work on a horse interesting and novel, to say the least. Being on television makes you a local celebrity and gives you publicity that exceeds the immediate viewing audience. Horse owners will find out about your interest in equine dentistry from their non–horse owning acquaintances who saw you on TV.

Getting exposure on television requires piquing the interest of someone in the broadcasting industry. This could be the person in charge of human-interest stories for your local news station or a local talk show host.

The human-interest angle is usually a spontaneous approach that is directed largely by the style and whimsy of the reporter, but you can control the situation to a certain extent. Arrange for the news team to videotape you working in a quiet, controlled environment on a gentle, predictable horse. Look professional. Wear a clean, pressed pair of coveralls. Explain to the reporter why regular dental care is so important for horses. Tell the reporter that horse's teeth erupt throughout life, and show them the oral pathology created by everyday wear. Be pleasant and personable. When they are finished videotaping you, thank them for their time and ask when the story will be on the air. Ask if you can get a copy. When it does air, expect the unexpected and keep your sense of humor. Most of what you say will be edited out—often to produce a short piece that is longer on humor than it is on education. But that doesn't matter. You will get your name associated with equine dentistry in a positive way in front of a wide audience.

The talk show is more formal and interview oriented. Be prepared. Watch an episode of the program before you appear on it so you can get a feel for the type of questions the interviewer asks. Sometimes you can give them a suggested list of questions to ask you. Rehearse beforehand by staging mock interviews using family, friends, or staff members as interviewers.

KEY POINT:
▶ Know what your main points are, and try to get them across early in the interview.

Find out what kind of visual aids you can use. Dress appropriately—if the interviewer always wears a suit, then, if you are a man, you should wear a jacket, tie, and nice slacks. If you are a woman, wear a business dress, or a skirt, etc. If the interviewer wears sweaters and corduroys, either sex would look professional in khaki slacks and a jacket. Ties for men are a must, even if the interviewer doesn't wear one. Finally, try to relax, listen closely to the questions, and answer them in a friendly, sincere manner in terms that the layperson can understand.

■ ■ SPECIAL EVENTS

KEY POINT:
▶ County, state, and regional fairs and horse expos are special events that welcome exhibitors with horse care information to share. Some horse shows and rodeos also have exhibit areas or trade shows associated with them.

Participating in a special event usually requires planning months or even a year in advance. To get started, contact the president or director of the board of the association producing the event. That person can tell you who is in charge of the event-planning committee. The planning committee can give you information about dates, costs, and reserving a booth. If your booth is promoting equine dental health education and not just your services, you may be able to get a complimentary booth. You can also ask your state veterinary association if it will sponsor the booth.

Decorate your booth in an eye-catching manner. A larger professionally made vinyl banner makes an inexpensive and reusable backdrop. You will need several tables, table skirts, and table covers. Find out if you have to rent these from the exhibit hall or if you are to provide your own. You will need a power outlet from the exhibit hall if you are going to have videotapes or slide monitors, lights, or demonstrations of dremel equipment. Bring your horse skulls, dental equipment, handouts, and books for sale. Set up a skull with your full-mouth speculum in it so you can demonstrate an examination. Don't forget comfort items for yourself and any helpers, such as a cooler of cold drinks, snacks, sandwiches, and chairs. Bring lots of enthusiasm. People are very curious about dentistry, so it may be a marathon of answering questions. One final note, don't ever leave your booth unattended, or you may lose a skull or equipment. If possible, always have another person to help you.

■ ■   PUBLIC SPEAKING

Even if you would rather have a root canal than speak in public, I encourage you to do it anyway. It is emotionally rewarding, especially when you have an audience that is hungry for information. Offer your services as a speaker to local riding clubs and 4-H groups. They are always looking for speakers and appreciate veterinarians who will take time to educate them about horse care. Organize your thoughts about the subject in a logical order so you don't have to speak from notes. Take your handouts and visual aids to reinforce your message. Relax and enjoy your role as information provider, and your audience will relax and won't notice if you are not the perfect public speaker.

PRACTICE TIP:
    Get information on giving effective presentations from books or videotapes. See the end of the chapter for a list of books.

■ ■   GET PUBLISHED

Writing articles is like public speaking. It is agonizing at first, but the more you do it, the easier it gets. Writing is less stressful than public speaking because you have the chance to review your article and keep changing it until you like it. But keep in mind that once it's in print, what you say is there for all the world to see and analyze, so make sure your information, grammar, spelling, and punctuation are correct. From a credibility point of view, getting your words in print is like being seen on television. It seems that if people in the media think you are worthy of being published, then you must be important. Be worthy of that credibility by writing informative, well-researched articles that focus on educating the public about equine dental abnormalities and the benefits of dentistry. Don't blow your own horn in the article, or your intentions may not appear to have the welfare of the horse as your primary interest, and don't claim you are a dental specialist unless you have the credentials to back it up. The most professional way to get credit for your knowledge is to ask the editor to include a byline at the bottom of the article: "Dr. X is an equine practitioner at ABC Equine Clinic and has a special interest in equine dentistry."

Publications you can contact about contributing articles to include local and regional horse magazines, agricultural newspapers and magazines, horse club newsletters, programs for horse shows and expos, and if you are feeling really brave, national horse magazines. Once you do get published, get lots of copies of the printed article, and don't be shy about handing them out during office calls, farm calls, and speaking engagements.

■ ■ **ADDITIONAL READING**

Beckwith H. Selling the Invisible: A Field Guide to Modern Marketing. New York: Warner Bros., 1997.

Toogood GN. The Articulate Executive: Learn to Look, Act, and Sound like a Leader. New York: McGraw-Hill, 1996.

Hoff R. I Can See You Naked. Andrews and McMeel: Kansas City, 1992.

GLOSSARY

Abrasion   the pathologic wearing away of a nonocclusal tooth surface or the oral mucosa.

Acute   sudden onset.

Alveolar Periostitis   inflammation of the periodontal tissues.

Alveolar Process   forms one-half of a dental arch (one-half of the upper or lower jaw).

Alveolus   the pit or socket that supports the individual tooth.

Ameloblasts   the dental cells that produce enamel.

Anachoretic Pulpitis   localized bacterial infection of the periapical region.

Apical   pertaining to the apex or tip of the tooth root.

Apical Foramen   the opening in the tooth root for the nerve, blood vessels, and lymphatics that supply the individual tooth.

Apicectomy   surgical removal of the apex of the tooth root.

Attrition   wearing away of the occlusal surface of the tooth by mastication.

Bacteremia   the usually transient condition of having bacteria in the circulating blood.

Bars   common term for the toothless area between the incisors and the cheek teeth in herbivores, the interdental space.

Beak   a descriptive term for a long, thin hook on a #06 tooth.

Bit Seat   the rostral corner of a #06 cheek tooth that has been rounded and smoothed for the comfort of the horse that carries a bit.

Blind Wolf Tooth   a fully erupted wolf tooth that has not penetrated the gingiva.

Bolus   a formed mass of chewed or partially chewed food.

Brachydont   teeth that have short crowns and long roots.

Brachygnathism   malocclusion in which the mandible is shorter than the maxilla; also called parrot mouth.

Bridle Tooth   common term for tooth #04. See Canine tooth.

Buccal   facing or pertaining to the mucous membrane on the inner surface of the cheek.

Calculus   concretion of minerals and organic material on the nonocclusal surface of teeth.

Canine Tooth   tooth #04. A curved and pointed tooth that functions to mortally wound prey or cause injury to opponents when fighting. The canine tooth has no masticatory function. Prominent canine teeth are found in male horses. Mares do not typically have canine teeth and when they do, they are usually small and undeveloped; also called a bridle tooth.

Cap   the deciduous tooth in which the root has been resorbed, leaving only the remnant of the reserve crown.

Carbide   a metal that has carbon added to increase its hardness, such as tungsten carbide.

Caries   decay of the organic components of dental tissue.

Caudal   the direction toward the posterior or tail end.

Cavesson   an adjustable noseband on the headstall of a bridle used for the purpose of preventing the horse from opening its mouth to escape the bit.

Cementoblasts   dental cells that produce cementum.

Cementoma   an uncommon reactive change occurring at the base of a developing tooth composed of cementum and fibrocellular tissues in varying proportions.

Cementum   the dull, yellowish external surface of the root and lining of the maxillary infundibula; composed of approximately 65% calcium hydroxyapatite (inorganic), 23% collagen fibers (organic), and 12% water.

Chronic   (in a disease) having long duration or recurring frequently.

Clubbing   descriptive term for the abnormal, blunted shape of a diseased tooth root as it appears radiographically.

Condition Score   a number assigned to an animal based upon the amount of flesh (fat) covering certain anatomical structures.

Coronal   the direction toward the crown of the tooth.

Crossfloat   a technique used in creating bit seats in which the float is introduced into the mouth and is used across the tongue, to float the tooth on the side opposite of the mouth. For example, in creating a bit seat on the #106 tooth (right side), the float is introduced through the interdental space on the left side, and the tooth is floated from the left side.

Crown   the portion of the tooth that is used for mastication.

Cribber   a horse that cribs.

Cribbing   a bad habit or vice in which the horse continually bites down hard on a solid object, which causes increased wear to the upper central incisors.

Cup   the deep, funnel-shaped depression in the center of an incisor tooth; the infundibulum of an incisor.

Curve of Spee   the rostral-caudal curve of the occlusal plane. The curve of the mandibular arch is concave; the curve of the maxillary arch is convex.

Cusp   an anatomical point or prominence on the crown of a tooth.

Dead Tooth   a nonscientific term referring to a tooth in a geriatric horse that has been worn to the dentin and cementum at the root end of the reserve crown where there is very little enamel; also can refer to a tooth that is no longer erupting.

Deciduous Tooth   one of the temporary teeth in a mammal that will be replaced by a permanent tooth; also called a baby tooth or a milk tooth.

Dental Arcade   the entire group of teeth of similar function in one side of the upper or lower jaw.

Dental Arch   the arch-shaped unit of bone that supports the teeth. The maxillary dental arch contains all of the upper teeth, and the mandibular dental arch contains all of the lower teeth.

Diagonal Bite   conformation of the incisors formed by abnormal attrition in which the incisal plane appears to be slanted when viewed from the front; also called a slant bite.

Diastema   the presence of a space between teeth; also called an interdental space.

Dominant Tooth   a nonscientific term that is sometimes used to refer to the longest tooth in a pair that is in occlusion. A dominant tooth may be created when one tooth erupts significantly earlier than the opposing tooth, which enables it to always be longer.

Dorsal Curvature   conformation of the incisors formed by abnormal attrition in which the lower central incisors are longer than the opposing upper incisors; may be seen in horses with oral vices such as cribbing or wind sucking; also called a frown confirmation.

Ear Tooth   a developmental anomaly in which dental tissue is found in areas of the head other than the jaws, most commonly in the temporal region near the ear.

Enamel   the hardest dental tissue and the hardest tissue in the body; composed of 95% hydroxyapatite crystals (inorganic tissue), 1% enamel matrix (organic tissue), and 4% water.

Eruption   the physiological movement of a tooth from the jaw into the oral cavity.

Eruption Cysts   swellings in the mandible or maxilla of a young horse associated with the osseous and vascular changes occurring during root formation and tooth eruption; also called pseudocysts.

Excessive Crown   a tooth having more exposed crown than the guide tooth in the arcade.

Excessive Transverse Ridges   excessive length of the transverse ridges created by the enamel foldings on the occlusal surfaces of the cheek teeth; also referred to as accentuated transverse ridges.

Fistula   a narrow tract usually created by an infectious process from the source of infection to the outer surface of the body.

Float   procedure that involves smoothing and leveling a rough surface. In equine dentistry, it refers to rasping off the sharp enamel points on the outer edges of the upper cheek teeth and the inner edges on the lower cheek teeth.

Frenulum   the central fold of mucosal tissue on the underside of the tongue.

Full Mouth   a horse in which all of the permanent teeth are erupted and in wear; an old term used to describe a horse as being 5 years old or older.

Gag   a simple device with no hinges used to hold open the jaws, usually inserted between the teeth on one side of the mouth.

Guide Tooth   the tooth in the arcade that is determined to have the most correct length. The height of the other teeth in that arcade will be evaluated by comparing them to the guide tooth.

Hook   a pointed, narrow protuberance off the rostral corner of a #06 tooth or the caudal corner of a #11 tooth created by overgrowth of a portion of occlusal surface that is not in occlusion.

Hypoplastic Cementum   condition in which there is inadequate formation of the cemental lake in the infundibulum in a maxillary cheek tooth. Incomplete filling of the infundibulum allows food and bacteria to accumulate, creating conditions conducive to caries formation.

Hypsodont   teeth having long crowns and short roots.

Impacted Tooth   tooth that cannot erupt normally due to overcrowding or abnormal position in the jaw.

Incisal   the occlusal surface of an incisor.

Incisor Alignment   the position of the incisal surfaces of the incisors relative to a level or horizontal plane.

Infraorbital Canal   the osseous canal that houses the infraorbital nerve and is intimately associated with the roots of maxillary teeth #08, 09, 10, and 11.

Infraorbital Nerve   a branch of the maxillary nerve that divides into branches that supply sensation to the upper lip and nostrils.

Infundibulum   the funnel-shaped, enamel-lined depression in an incisor tooth and maxillary cheek tooth. Incisors have one infundibulum; maxillary cheek teeth have two infundibuli.

Interdental Space   the space between teeth; also used to describe the toothless area that separates the incisors and the cheek teeth.

Labial   direction toward the lips or the tooth surface of an incisor tooth that faces the lips.

Lamina Dura   the thin, hard layer of bone that lines the alveolus of a tooth.

Lampas   swelling of the hard palate thought to be associated with tooth eruption found just caudal to the upper incisors.

Lateral Excursion   the side-to-side movement of the mandible.

Lesion   a well-defined abnormal change created by disease or injury to tissue.

Lingual   the direction toward the tongue, or the tooth surface of a mandibular tooth that faces the tongue.

Loph   the portion of an enamel fold of a tooth that defines a transverse ridge.

Lysis   disintegration or dissolution of cells.

Maldigestion   impaired or inadequate digestion.

Marginal   toward or pertaining to the area of gingiva where it interfaces with a tooth.

Median   the line that separates the right side of the body from the left side.

Mesial   the surface of a tooth that is closest to the front of the mouth.

Molarization the evolutionary change of premolar teeth into teeth that are indistinguishable from molars.

Monkey Mouth undershot jaw. *See* prognathism.

Nasomaxillary Aperature the opening between the rostral maxillary sinus and the middle nasal meatus or passage.

Nasopharynx the upper part of the oral cavity that is continuous with the nasal passages.

Necrotic decayed or decomposed.

Necrotic Infundibulum a term incorrectly used to describe caries of the infundibulum of a maxillary cheek tooth.

Neoplastic new growth of tissue that serves no physiological purpose. Used to describe a tumor or a cancerous lesion.

Occlusion the relationship or contact between surfaces of teeth opposing each other in the upper and lower jaws.

Odontoblasts dental cells that secrete dentin.

Orthodontic pertaining to abnormalities of tooth and/or jaw position.

Palatal the direction toward the palate or the surface of a maxillary tooth that faces the palate.

Parrot Mouth *see* brachygnathism.

Periodontal Ligament the fibrous tissue that connects the cementum of a tooth root to the alveolus.

Periodontium the supporting structures of the teeth, including the alveolus, the periodontal ligament, the cementum, and the associated gingiva.

Periostitis inflammation of the periodontal structures.

Plaque the film of bacteria-harboring mucus and organic material that covers the tooth.

Polydontia developmental abnormality in which there are more teeth present than predicted by the dental formula for the species.

Primary Dentin the dentin that is formed as a part of normal tooth development.

Prognathism developmental orthodontic abnormality in which the lower jaw is longer than the upper jaw.

Proximal the surface of a tooth that faces another tooth.

Pulp the soft tissues within the center of the tooth. The dental pulp has four important functions: 1. Formative—the pulp contains odontoblasts, the dentin-forming cells that produce dentin throughout the life of the tooth. 2. Sensory—nerves in the pulp allow sensation of pain, heat, cold, and pressure. 3. Nutritive—nutrients are transported to the odontoblasts in the blood vessels in the pulp. 4. Protection—the odontoblasts in the pulp respond to injury by forming reparative dentin.

Ramp the abnormal attrition of a tooth in which the tooth is worn to a ramp-like appearance, i.e., one end of the tooth is taller (longer) than the other; usually refers to a #06 or a #11 tooth.

Recessed Crown   exposed crown of a cheek tooth that is shorter than the guide tooth.

Reduce   to remove tooth material.

Reparative Dentin   dentin formed in response to tooth injury to seal the pulp from exposure to the oral cavity.

Repulsion   to extract a cheek tooth by pushing it out of the socket into the oral cavity through a surgically created opening in the jaw bone, using a dental punch placed against the tooth roots that is struck with a mallet.

Reserve Crown   the portion of the crown of a hypsodont tooth that is below the gingiva.

Resorption   the process of being broken down and assimilated, as in the resorption of the root of a deciduous tooth.

Rim   a thin line of enamel on the occlusal surface of a tooth.

Rongeur   surgical instrument used to remove small pieces of bone.

Rostral   the direction toward the front of an animal; also called anterior.

Sagittal   a line down the median dividing the body or a part (i.e., tooth) into unequal right and left parts.

Sclerosis   pathological hardening of a tissue.

Secondary Dentin   dentin produced in response to a chronic irritation, such as attrition to the occlusal surface of a tooth.

Sharpey's Fibers   connective tissue fibers in the periosteum that connect tendon to bone by penetrating into the cortex of the bone.

Shear Mouth   a sharp, exceedingly slanted occlusal surface (table angle greater than 15 degrees) that produces an excessively long buccal aspect to the upper cheek teeth and lingual aspect of the lower cheek teeth. Shear mouth can be seen in horses with abnormally narrow mandibles, horses with mandibular injuries, or horses in which mastication has been so painful for a long period of time that mastication is primarily performed in an up-and-down, not side-to-side, manner.

Smooth Mouth   a horse in which all of the incisor teeth have worn so that there are no cups or infundibuli present in the incisal surface; an old term used to describe a horse that is past a certain age, usually 12 years or older.

Speculum   an instrument used to widen a body orifice for the purpose of visual inspection, delivery of medication, or performance of a procedure.

Squiffy Nose   descriptive term describing the congenital lateral deviation of the rostral portion of the nose; also called wry nose.

Standard System   method of numbering the teeth of the horse in which each tooth is identified by a capital letter(s) depicting what type of tooth it is (I = incisor, PM = premolar, M = molar) and a number assigning its position in the mouth relative to the median line.

Step Mouth   abrupt variation in the height of adjacent teeth caused by abnormal eruption or missing teeth.

Stomatitis inflammation of the oral cavity.

Sulcus furrow or groove. In teeth, a groove on a nonocclusal surface of a cheek tooth formed by folding of the enamel.

Super-Erupting Tooth a term sometimes used to describe a tooth that is longer than its counterpart in the opposite arcade.

Table Angle the angle of the occlusal surface of a cheek tooth when compared to a level or horizontal surface.

Tartar *see* calculus.

Tertiary Dentin another term for reparative dentin; dentin formed in response to injury of a tooth.

Transverse Ridges ridges on the occlusal surface of a cheek tooth created by attrition of the tooth surface around the enamel lophs.

Trephine a hole drilled through a bone in the skull. In horses, it is usually a hole drilled or punched into a sinus.

Triadan System system for numbering teeth that divides the mouth into quadrants that specify whether the tooth is in the upper or lower jaw and whether it is on the right or left side (1 = upper right, 2 = upper left, 3 = lower left, 4 = lower right). The individual teeth are then numbered according to their position relative to the median line, starting with the central incisor in the quadrant.

Ventral Curvature smile conformation of the incisors; the incisor conformation created by wear on the increasingly rostral angulation of the incisors as they erupt by the rotational mastication pattern used in herbivores to grind roughage.

Vestigial a small, undeveloped body part that may have had a function in an ancestral form of an animal.

Wave Complex a group of cheek teeth in an arcade in which the varying heights form a wave.

Wave Mouth a term describing an abnormality of attrition in which the occlusal surface of the cheek teeth has an undulating appearance.

Wolf Tooth tooth #05, the first premolar; thought to be a vestigial tooth.

Wry Nose congenital lateral deviation of the rostral portion of the nose.

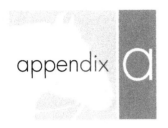

appendix a

EQUINE DENTAL EQUIPMENT AND INSTRUMENT SUPPLIERS

Alberts Dental Supply
336 Loudon Road
Loudonville, NY 12211
1-800-DENTAL-8

Brassler USA Inc. Dental Instruments
800 King George Blvd.
Savannah, GA 31419
1-800-841-4522

Capps Manufacturing
4804 W. Birch
Clatonia, NE 68328
402-989-4022

Carbide Products Company
Equine Division
22711 S. Western Avenue
Torrance, CA 90501
310-320-7910

Conrad Full-Mouth Speculum
Harold Conrad
352-429-3808

D & B Equine Enterprises Inc.
207 Silverhill Way
N.W. Calgary, Alberta
Canada T3B 4K9
403-615-2661
www.powerfloat.com

DLM Tool Works
P.O. Box 457
Simonton, TX 77476
281-346-2355 or 281-533-9699

Dremel
4915 21st St.
Racine, WI 53406
1-800-4-DREMEL

Enco Machinery, Tools and Supplies
1-800-873-3626

Equi-Dent Technologies
P.O. Box 5877
Sparks, NV 89432
702-358-6695

Equine Veterinary Dental Instruments
8456 East Highway 24
Manhattan, KS 66502
913-537-9559

Harlton's Equine Specialties
792 Olenhurst Court
Columbus, OH 43235-2163
1-800-247-3901

Jorgensen Laboratories
1450 N. Van Buren
Loveland, CO 80538
303-669-2500

Jupiter Veterinary Products
4504 Lakeside Drive
Harrisburg, PA 17110
717-233-6131

Lang Dental Manufacturing Company
2300 W. Wabonsia Avenue
Chicago, IL 60647
Fax: 312-486-0107

Milburn Distributions
P.O. Box 42810
Phoenix, AZ 85308
800-279-6452

Olsen and Silk Abrasives
35 Congress Street, Building 2
Salem, MA 01970
508-744-4720

Promax Equine Dental
1-800-933-1562

Rach Holdings
35 Silvergrove Court NW
Calgary, Alberta
Canada T3B 5A3
403-286-5256

Stubbs Equine Innovations
HC3, Box 38
Johnson City, TX 78636
830-868-7544

Swissvet Veterinary Products LLC
1952 Lee Rd. 65
Auburn, AL 36830
1-877-773-5628
www.swissvet.com

Western Instrument Company
4950 York Street
P.O. Box 16428
Denver, CO 80216
1-800-525-2065

World Wide Equine
P.O. Box 1040
Glenns Ferry, ID 83623
1-800-331-5485

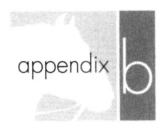

appendix b

Spare parts commonly needed for Dremel instruments (1-800-4-DREMEL).

Model 235 Handpiece (small handpiece)
    Collet nut—part #5294093
    $\frac{1}{8}''$ collet—part #480
    Ball—part #350998
    Spring clip—part #5295081
    Wrench—part #90962

Model 236 Handpiece (large handpiece)
    Collet nut—part #5295090
    $\frac{1}{4}''$ collet—part #590
    Spring washer—part #68894
    Bearing and shaft assembly—part #5295083
    Boot (heel of hand piece)—part #5295082
    Ball—part #350998
    Spring clip—part #5295081
    Wrench—part #5295097
    Pin—part #5295096

Heavy-Duty Flex-Shaft Tool Model #732
    Foot speed control—part #221
    Table-top speed control—part #219
    Cable—part #5295052
    Flexible shaft grease—part #90952
    Casing assembly for cable—part #5295051

INDEX

Page numbers in italics denote figures; those followed by a t denote tables; those followed by a b denote boxes.